MW00582811

PATHOGENESIS
IN
AYURVEDA
(SAMPRAPTI)

THE
CHAUKHAMBA AYURVIJNAN STUDIES
17

PATHOGENESIS
IN
AYURVEDA
(SAMPRAPTI)

Dr. V. B. Athavale
M.D., D. C. H., M. A. M. S.
Vaidyacharya

CHAUKHAMBA SANSKRIT PRATISHTHAN

DELHI

PATHOGENESIS IN AYURVEDA

Publishers

© CHAUKHAMBA SANSKRIT PRATISHTHAN

38 U. A. Bungalow Road, Jawahar Nagar
Delhi 110007
Phone : (011) 23856391, 41530902
e-mail : csp_praveen@rediffmail.com

All Rights Reserved

Reprinted : 2009
ISBN : 81-7084-140-2
Price : Rs. 350.00

Also can be had from
CHOWKHAMBA VIDYABHAWAN
Chowk (Behind Bank of Baroda Building)
Post Box. No. 1069
Varanasi 221001

CHAUKHAMBA SURBHARATI PRAKASHAN
K. 37/117 Gopal Mandir Lane
Post Box. No. 1129
Varanasi 221001

CHAUKHAMBA PUBLISHING HOUSE
4697/2, Ground Floor, Street No. 21-A
Ansari Road, Darya Ganj
New Delhi 110002

Printers
A. K. Lithographers, Delhi

Dedicated
to
The Research Workers
of
Past, Present & Future

ACKNOWLEDGEMENTS

I am grateful to my teacher Vaidya Venimadhava Shastri Joshi for giving me insight in pathogenesis of diseases. I am thankful to Dr. Sanjay Javale, Dr. Suresh Maroli and Dr. Sankanur Rao for their untiring help.

*O Lord ! you are the creator of the entire universe,
You have cursed the living creatures by creating
diseases, so that, they are punished for their sins
of the present as well as of past lives. I request
you to pardon all the creatures for all their sins
by giving an insight to physicians about root,
causes and evolution of diseases, so that they can
eardicate and prevent each and every disease*

त्वमेव भगवान् हेतुर्विश्वोत्पत्ते: प्रकीर्तित:।
स्वकर्मफलभोगाय रोगाणामपि कारक:।।
दयाक्षमादिगुणवान् त्वमेवासि न चापर:।
रोगोत्पत्तिनिदानादि ज्ञानं सम्यक् प्रदीयताम्।।
चिकित्सकेभ्य: सर्वेभ्यो दयासंसूचकं तव।
येन सर्वेऽपि भिषजो निदानादि चिकित्सितम्।।
विधाय सम्यगगदान् करिष्यन्ति जनान् पुन:।
अपुनर्भवाय सर्वेऽपि नशिष्यन्ति यथा गदा:।।
तवानुकम्पयैवैतत्सर्वं सिद्धं भविष्यति।
अत: सम्प्रार्थयामि त्वाम् अनुकम्पां विधेहि भो:।।

PREFACE

Pathogenesis deals with evolution of disease. It deals with, (i) various aetiological factors, (ii) how the aetiological factors bring about changes in the structural and functional units of the body, i.e. *Vata, Pitta* and *Kapha*, (iii) how these molecular changes bring about structural derangement in various tissues and organs, (iv) how these structural changes derange the function of organs, and (v) how the deranged function of one organ leads to derangement of other organs, i.e. complications.

Ayurveda describes in detail the various stages of evolution of disease as (i) *Chaya,* i.e. accumulation of *doshas* because of action of aetiological factors, (ii) *Prakopa,* i.e. further increase in the *doshas,* (iii) *Prasara,* i.e. dissemination of *doshas* which correspond to the stage of septicemia, viremia or toxaemia, (iv) *Sthanasanshraya,* i.e. localisation of *dosha* in a particular tissue or organ, (v) *Vyakti,* i.e. manifestation of disease because of functional derangement, and (vi) *Bheda,* i.e. further differentiation into the sub-type of the disease.

Ayurveda emphasises that the physician should not allow the disease to evolve further by recognising manifestations of the disease in its incubation period and guiding the patient appropriately. It is surprising that even 5,000 years ago, Ayurvedic physicians could visualise the derangement at molecular level as the root cause of the disease. Ayurveda has rightly emphasised on the importance of understanding the pathogenesis, i.e. evolution of disease. Unless the physician gets insight into the pathogenesis of the diseases, he cannot treat the patient appropriately. A physician who does not bother to go to the root cause of the disease suppresses the symptoms but is unable to eradicate the disease. This book describes in detail the basic principles of pathogenesis which will help the reader to understand the pathogenesis of any symptom or disease.

One can't but appreciate the wisdom of out ancient physicians, when one realises that our understanding of disease process and its evolution has not altered significantly even today, inspite of all the modern research. I am sure that not only Ayurvedic physicians but also students, teachers and research workers of modern medicine also will be benefited by this book.

V. B. Athavale

CONTENTS

1
DISEASE
ITS ORIGIN AND CLASSIFICATION
(ROGANAM UTPATTI VIBHAGASHCHA)

The unbalanced state of tissue, *doshas* and waste products is defined as disease, whereas their balanced state is termed as health. Health is happiness, whereas disease is sorrow. When the *dhatus*, *doshas* or *malas* are affected by increased, decreased or abnormal *doshas*, the disease sets in.

The word disease is derived from *dis* and *ease* meaning disturbance of ease. The synonyms of disease in Ayurveda are :

(1) The words *roga*, *vyadhi*, *dukha* and *abadha* all of which are synonyms of the word disease, which means pain or sorrow.

(2) *Papma*, i.e. one which arises as a result of sins.

(3) *Amaya* is one which arises as a result of indigestion.

(4) *Vikara* is one which is associated with disturbed structure or functions of various organs.

(5) *Jvara* is one which is associated with fever and irritability of mind.

(6) *Yakshma*, i.e. one which is associated with wasting.

(7) *Atanka* is one which is associated with unbearable state.

(8) *Gada*, i.e. one which can arise from various aetiological factors.

ORIGIN OF DISEASES

In the begining of *Satya-yuga*, men were endowed with vitality equal to that of God's. Exceedingly faultless and unhampered in their powers, they had direct knowledge of Gods. The God like sages knew the divine law, and the sacrificial rituals. They possessed body which were compact and firm and had clear sense and mind. They had good complexion and their speed, strength and power resembled those of the wind. They were free from fear, desire, aversion, infactuation, greed, anger, pride, diseases, laziness, fatigue, languour and the spirit of acquisition. They were endowed with unlimited longevity. For the benefit of these people of heroic minds, qualities and deeds, the crops were replete with wonderful taste, potency, post digestive effect, specific action and virtue, as the earth during the dawn of the golden age was charged to the full with all excellent qualities.

During later part of *Krita-yuga* or *Satya-yuga*, those who were better financially ate more and became obese. By over-indulgence this heaviness of body bred lassitude, lassitude gave rise to indolence, indolence created the need of accumulation and necessitated acquisition. The spirit of acquisition engendered greed. The qualities of earth also deteriorated gradually along with the qualities of man.

Thereafter, the bodies of human beings failing to receive nutrition as before from the progressively deterioration quality of food along with lack of exercise and adverse effects of exertion, heat and wind, soon succumbed to attacks of fever and other disease. Thus, there was a gradual decline in the life span enjoyed by successive generations. Thereafter, in the second or silver age, i.e. *Treta-yuga*, greed brought malice in its way and led to false-hood, falsehood let loose lust, anger, vanity, hatred, cruelty, aggression, fear grief, anxiety, distress and the like. Consequently in the second age, virtue found itself deprived of a quarter of its plentitude. From this quarterly loss in virtue, there followed a similar deterioration in the duration of the succeeding age and in the beneficient power of the earth and other elements. It is in consequence of this deterioration that there took place a corres-ponding deterioration in the purity, taste, potency, post-digestive effects, specific action and quality of herbs. In this manner righteousness dwindled in each succeeding age by one quarter and the proto-elements too suffered similar deterioration till eventually the world would come to dissolution.

When a hunderedth part of the length of an age period is past, then the life span of creatures gets less by one year. This is said with reference to the normal determination of life span in a given age. Thus, not following the path of righteousness and not following the dictates of conscience are the root cause of all the diseases.

CLASSIFICATION OF DISEASES

Diseases are classified in various ways as follows :

(i) *Diseases of Body and Mind* : It is based on whether the disease affects the body or mind. Increase, decrease or vitiation of *doshas, dhatus* and *malas* gives rise to diseases of body. The root causes of mental diseases are non-fulfillment of one's desires and presence of unpleasant situations. These factors increase *raja* and *tama* qualities of mind. The increased *raja* gives rise to emotional upsets such as anger, sorrow, jealousy, hatred and greed. The increased *tama* gives rise to laziness, ignorance, inability to take decisions and unclear thoughts. The increased *raja* and *tama*, in turn disturb *Vata, Pitta* and *Kapha doshas* and gives rise to mental as well as psychosomatic illnesses.

(ii) *Nija and Agantu Diseases* : The word *nija* means self. The root cause of all *nija*, i.e. self induced diseases is not following the dictates of one's conscience. The indiscretions in diet and activities disturb the balance of *Vata, Pitta* and *Kapha* and give rise to various illness.

These diseases are caused by external factors like injury, burns, accidental poisoning, exposure to cyclones, lightening and earthquakes, bites of animals and insects, invasion of body by germs and supernatural powers like ghosts, curses etc. In *agantu* diseases, the tissues or organs are affected first and the balance of *doshas* is disturbed later.

(iii) *Ekadoshaja, Dvandvaja and Sannipatika Diseases* : The diseases are classified according to the number of *doshas* affected. In *ekadoshaja* disease, only one *dosha* is affected. In *dvandvaja* two *doshas* are affected, while in *sannipatika* diseases all the three *doshas* are affected. The increase in various *doshas* may be mild, moderate or severe. Depending on the permutations and combinations of the degrees of rise in various *doshas*, one gets twenty five types of *sannipatika*, e. g. in *ekolbana sannipata*, one *doshas* is very much increased, whereas other *doshas* are only slightly increased. Similarly, all the three *doshas* may be decreased in varying degrees. Also in *hinamadhyadhika sannipata*, one *dosha* is slightly increased, second *dosha* is moderately increased, while third *dosha* is very much increased.

(iv) *Sushruta's Classification* :

  (a) Hereditary diseases *(Adibala pravritta* or *sahaja* diseases)*—These diseases arise due to defective chromosomes or genes transmitted from father or mother.

  (b) Congenital diseases *(Janmabala pravritta* or *garbhaja* diseases)—These diseases are caused by charomosomal or genetic anomalies. In addition, various factors operating on the foetus in the intra-uterine life also lead to congenital diseases, e. g. indiscretion in diet or activity of mother, effects of drugs taken by mother, disease in mother, etc.

  (c) Diseases caused by *doshas (Doshabala pravritta* or *jataja* diseases)—Disturbances in *Vata*, *Pitta* and *Kapha* takes place as a result of indiscretion in diet and activity, which can affect both body as well as mind. They are further classified as diseases due to increased *dosha* or decreased *dosha*.

  (d) Traumatic diseases *(Sanghata-bala pravritta* or *pida-krita)*—These traumatic diseases can be classified further as physical trauma, e.g. injuries, accidents, operations, etc. and mental traumae, e.g. sudden unexpected bad news, sudden loss of money, etc.

(e) Diseases due to environmental factors (*Kala-bala pravritta* or *kalaja* diseases)—The Various environmental factors like heat, cold and exposure to rain also lead to diseases. They can be further classified as :

    (i) Diseases due to seasonal changes, i.e. *avyapanna rhitu-krita,* and

    (ii) Diseases due to sudden unexpected changes in the environment, i.e. *vyapanna-rhitu-krita.*

(f) Diseases arising due to bad luck or misfortune (*Daiva-bala pravritta* or *prabhavaja* diseases)—These diseases arise, when one insults teachers, parents, respected people or God or due to one's bad deeds either in this or past lives. They also can arise as a result of affection by supernatural powers like ghosts or curses of sages.

(g) Natural disease (*Svabhava-bala pravritta*) — These are hunger, sleep, thirst, old age and death. They are also further classified as :

    (i) *Kala-krita* or timely diseases, i.e. when they occur expectedly, and

    (ii) *Akala-krita* or Untimely diseases, i.e. when they occur unexpectedly.

(v) *Diseases of Tissues, Associated Tissues and Waste Products* : Diseases of tissues, i.e. *dhatu,* associated tissues, i.e. *upadhatu* and waste products, i.e. *mala.*

(vi) *Diseases According to the State of Nutrition* :

(a) *Santarpa-nottha* diseases, i.e. diseases due to over nutrition, e.g. obesity, diabetes. Eating oily, fatty, sweet and heavy food items like meat of aquatic animals, jaggery, starch in excess, sleeping during the day and leading an inactive life leads to overnutrition and various diseases associated with it. These diseases are obesity, diabetes, diabetic skin lesions, skin disorders of *Kaphaja* type, itching, anaemia, fever, diseases associated with *ama* dysuria, laziness, drowsiness, heaviness, feeling as if *Kapha* is sticking to various body channels and sense and motor organs, giddiness, worry and oedema.

(b) *Apatarpanottha vyadhi,* i. e. diseases due to under-nutrition, e.g. emaciation, tuberculosis. Taking dry, light and inadequate quantity of food, fasting and excessive exertion lead to diseases associated with under-nutrition. Under-nutrition leads to loss of weight and strength, weak digestive power, wasting of all the tissues, loss of lustre of the skin, fever with cough, pleural effusion, loss of taste sensation, impaired hearing, delirium, insanity, heart disease, constipation, oliguria, pain in the thighs, sacrum and joints and all varieties of *Vataja* diseases.

(vii) *Prakriti-Sama-Samavaya and Vikriti-Vishama Samavaya* : Diseases caused by two or more *doshas,* i.e. *dvandvaja* or *sannipatika* are classified into *prakriti-sama-samavaya* and *vikriti-vishama-samavaya.*

In *prakriti-sama-samavya* type, the manifestations of increased *doshas* are encountered as expected. In *vikriti-vishama-samavaya* apart from the expected manifestations, one also gets unexpected manifestations. This may be explained on the assumption that *prakriti-sama-samavaya* represents the simultaneous affection of two or more *doshas,* were are the *vikriti-vishama-samavaya* represents chemical combination of two or more *doshas.*

(viii) *Major and Minor Diseases* : *Mahagada,* i.e. major diseases are difficult to cure, tend to become chronic or produce unbearable pain or are associated with high mortality.

(a) *Vatavyadhi,* i.e. diseases of nervous system,

(b) *Apasmara,* i.e. epilepsy,

(c) Major skin diseases,

(d) *Prameha* and *Madhumeha*, i.e. metabolic disorders with characteristic urinary abnormality and diabetes mellitus,

(e) *Udara*, i.e. enlargement of abdomen due to ascites,

(f) *Shotha*, i.e. generalised anasarca,

(g) *Rajayakshma*, i.e. tuberculosis,

(h) *Gulma*, i.e. tumour arising as a result of weakness of wall of an organ,

(i) *Ashmari*, i.e. calculi, e.g. renal or gall stones,

(j) *Bhagandara*, i.e. fistula in ano,

(k) *Arsha*, i.e. piles,

(l) *Grahani*, i.e. malabsorption syndrome, and

(m) *Mudhagarbha*, i.e. abnormal presentation of foetus.

These major diseases are often associated with some complication like lack of vitality, emaciation, hiccup, breathlessness, thirst, vomiting, fever fainting, diarrhoea, etc.

(ix) *Disease According to Region of the Body Affected* : According to the region of the body affected, diseases are classified as peripheral diseases, diseases of middle zone and diseases of digestive tract.

(a) *Diseases of peripheral structures* : These are classified as : (i) Skin diseases, (ii) Disorders of body fluid, and (iii) Blood disorders.

(b) *Diseases of middle zone* : These are classified as : (i) Diseases of nervous system, (ii) Diseases of genito-urinary system, (iii) Cardio-vascular diseases, (iv) Respiratory diseases, and (v) Musculo-skeletal diseases.

(c) *Diseases of the digestive tract* : It includes diseases of gastro-intestina tract, liver, spleen and pancreas.

(x) *Anubandhi Doshas and Diseases (Anubandhya)* : A disease may arise as a result of simultaneous increase of one, two or all the three doshas. These are termed as *Kevala*, *Dvandvaja* or *Tridoshaja* disease, e.g. when cough starts due to simultaneous increase in both *Pitta* and *Kapha*, it is termed as *Pitta-kaphaja kasa*. When cough starts dtie to market increase in *Pitta* and slight increase in *Kapha*, it is termed as *Sakapha-pittaja kasa*. When cough due to increased *Kapha*, i.e. *Kaphaja kasa* is followed by increased *Pitta* and aggravates the original disease, it is termed as *pittanubandhikaphaja kasa*.

(xi) *Pachanatmaka, Shodhanalmaka and Prachayatmaka Diseases* : Some authors classify the diseases according to their pathogenesis. In any disease the *doshas* accumulate, increase, spread, get localized in a particular organ and lead to mani-festations of diseases after damaging the organ. The body tries to decrease the *doshas* by : (a) digestion of the *doshas* , i.e. *pachana*, (b) by getting rid of *doshas* from the body, i.e. *shodhana,* and (c) by localisation and accumulation of *doshas* in one part of the body, i.e. *prachayatmaka.*

According to the dominant defence mechanism of the body, the discascs are classified as *pachanatmaka, shodhanatmaka* and *prachayatmaka.*

Pachantmaka diseases : Fever, abscesses and all infections and inflammatory diseases represent *pachanatmaka* diseases. In these diseases, body tries to neutralise and decrease the accumu-lated *doshas* by their digestion through tissue enzymes.

Shodhanatmaka disease : Diseases like vomiting, cold, cough etc. in which the body tries to get rid off *doshas* through natural passages are termed as *shodhanatmaka* diseases. In these diseases, one should not try to suppress the natural passage of toxins in early stages of the disease.

Prachayatmaka diseases : If the rate of accumulation of *doshas* exceeds that of digestion or removal of the *doshas*, the result is *prachayatmaka* diseaes.Various tumors, enlargement of glands, hypertrophy of various organs, hepato-splenomegaly, obesity, etc. are some of the examples of *prachayatmaka* diseases.

These diseases usually manifest slowly and the symptoms manifest late. The patient gets gradually adapted to the slowly accumulating *doshas*. By promoting local accumulation of *doshas*, body tries to prevent dissemination and damage to other organs.

Thus, diseases can be classified in many ways. The above mentioned classification gives clue to understanding the various aspects of diseases.

रोगाणाम् उत्पत्ति:विभागश्च

व्याधय:

विविधं दु:खं आदधति इति व्याधि: प्रायेण आमसमुत्थत्वेनामय इत्युच्यते।

(च. नि. टीका)

पापस्य कर्मण: फलमिति पाप्मा। बुद्धीन्द्रियमन:

शरीराणां विकृतिमन्ययातं जनयति इति विकार:

यक्ष्मा इव यक्ष्मा। यथा यक्ष्मा रोगसमूहाणाभित्युक्तम्।

एषं सर्वेंऽपि रोग: रोगसमूह: इत्यनेन द्योतयति तथा च

सर्वे विकारा उत्पहमाना अनेकैर्व्याधिलक्षणै: उत्पद्यन्ते।

कृच्छ्रजीवने इत्यस्य धातो: रूपं आतङ्क इति।

यज्जीवति तन्मरणं यन्मरणं सोऽस्य विश्राम:।

गद इव गद: अनेककारणनन्यत्वात्।

आ समन्तात् कायमनसो: बाधनं पीडा इति आबाध:।

ज्वरयति इति ज्वर: ज्वरयति संतापयति।

आगन्तुर्न्वेति निज विकारं निजस्तथाऽऽगन्तुमपिप्रवृद्ध:। (च. सू. 19/7)

व्याधि पर्याया:

तत्र व्याधिरमय: गद आतङ्को यक्ष्मा ज्वरो रोग इत्यनर्थान्तरम्। (च. नि. 1/5)

रोग: पाप्मा ज्वरो व्याधिर्विकारो दु:खमामय:।

यक्ष्मातङ्कगदाबाधा: शब्दा: पर्यायवाचिन:। (अ. ह्र. नि. 1/1)

व्याधि प्रकारा:

त्रयो रोगा इति–निजागन्तुमानसा:। तत्र निज: शारीरदोषसमुत्थ:, आगन्तुर्भूतविषवाय्व-ग्निसम्प्रहारादिसमुत्थ: मानस: पुनरिष्टस्यालाभाल्लाभाच्चानिष्टस्योपजायते।

(च.सू. 11/45)

रोगोत्पत्तिः

आदिकाले ह्यदितिमुतसमौजसोऽतिविमलविपुलप्रभावाः प्रत्यक्षदेवदेवर्षिधर्मयज्ञ-
विधिविधानाः शैलसारसंहतस्थिरशरीराः प्रसन्नवर्णेन्द्रियाः पवनसमबलजवपराक्रमाः-
श्चारुस्फिचोऽभिरूपप्रमाणाकृतिप्रसादोपचयवन्तः सत्यार्जवानृशंस्यदानदमनियम-
तपउपवासब्रह्मचर्यव्रतपरा व्यपगतभयरागद्वेषमोहलोभक्रोधशोकमानरोगनिद्रातन्द्रा-
श्रमक्लमालस्यपरिग्रहाश्च पुरुषारबभूवुमुमितायुषः। तेषामुदारसत्त्वगुणकर्मणाम-
चिन्त्यरसवीर्यविपाकप्रभावगुणसमुदितानि प्रादुर्बभूवुःशस्यानि सर्वगुणसमुदितत्वात्,
पृथिव्यादीनां कृतयुगस्यादौ। भ्रश्यति तु कृतयुगे केषाञ्चिदित्यादानात् साम्पन्निकानां
सत्त्वानां शरीरगौरवमासीत्, शरीरगौरवाच्छ्रमः, श्रमादालस्यम्, आलस्यात् सञ्चयः,
सञ्चयात् परिग्रहः, परिग्रहाल लोभः प्रादुरासीत्कृते।

तत स्त्रेतायां लोभादभिद्रोहः, अभिद्रोहादनृतवचनम्, अनृतवचनात् कामक्रोधधमा-
नद्वेषपारुष्याभिघातभयतापशोकचिन्तोद्वेगादयः प्रवृत्ताः। ततस्त्रेतायां धर्मपादोऽन्त-
र्धानमगमत्। तस्यान्तर्धानाद् युगवर्षप्रमाणस्य पादह्रासः पृथिव्यादेश्च गुणपाद-
प्रणाशोऽभूत्। तत्प्रणाशकृतश्च शस्यानां स्नेहवैमल्यरशवीर्यविपाकप्रभावगुणपादभ्रंश।
ततस्तानि प्रजाशरीराणि हीयमानगुणपादैरहारविहारैर यथापूर्वमुपष्टभ्यमानान्यग्नि-
मारुतपरीतानि प्राग्व्याधिभि ज्वरादिभिराक्रान्तानि। अतः प्राणिनो ह्रासमवापुरायुषः
क्रमशः इति।

(च. वि. 3/24)

युगेयुगे धर्मपादः क्रमेणानेन हीयते।

गुणपाशच भूतानामेवंलोक: प्रलीयते।।

संवत्सरशतेपूर्णे याति संवत्सरः क्षयम्।

देहिनामायुषः काले यत्र यन्मानमिष्यते।।

इति विकाराणां प्रागुत्पत्तिहेतुरुक्तो भवति।। (च. वि. 3/25-27)

सुश्रुतोक्त-व्याधिप्रकारः

तत्तु सप्तविधे व्याधावुपनिपतति। ते पुनः सप्तविधा व्याधयः तद्यथा-
आदिबलप्रवृत्ताः, जन्मबलप्रवृत्ता दोषबलप्रवृत्ताः, संघात बलप्रवृत्ताः, दैवबलप्रवृत्ताः
स्वभावबलप्रवृत्ता इति।

तत्र आदिबलप्रवृत्ताः ये शुक्रशोणिदोषन्वया: कुष्ठार्श प्रभूतयः, तेऽपि
द्विविधाः- मातृजाः, पितृः च, जन्मबलप्रवृत्ता ये-मातुरुपचारात् पंगुजात्यन्धबधिरमूक-
मिन्मिन वामन प्रभृतयो जायन्तेः तेऽपि द्विविधाः, रसकृतः दौहृदापचार कृताश्च।

दोषबलप्रवृत्ता ये-आतकसमुत्पन्ना मिथ्याहाराचार कृताश्च, तेऽपि द्विविधा:, आमाशयसमुत्था: पक्वाशय समुत्थाश्च।

पुनश्चद्विविध:, शारीर, मानसश्च त, एते अध्यात्मिका:।

संघातबलप्रवृत्ता ये, आगन्तवो दुर्बलस्य, बलवद्विग्रहात्, तेऽपि द्विविधा:, शस्त्रकृता, व्यालकृताश्च। एते आदिभौतिका:।

कालबलप्रवृत्ताये शीतोष्णवातवर्षाप्रभृतिनिमिता:, तेऽपि द्विविधा:, व्यापन्न-ऋतुकृता अव्यापन्नऋतुकृताश्च, दैवबलप्रवृत्ताये देवद्रोहादभिशप्तका अथर्वणकृता उपसर्गजाश्च, तेऽपि द्विविधा:, विद्युदशनीकृता:, पिशाचविकृताश्च, पुनश्च द्विविधा:, संसर्गजा, आकस्मिकाश्च, स्वभावबलप्रवृत्ता: क्षुत्पिपासा जरामृत्युनिद्राप्रभृतय:, तेऽपि द्विविधा: कालकृता, अकालकृताश्च, तत्र परिरक्षणकृता अकालकृता:। एते आधिदैविका:। अत्र सर्व व्याधि अवरोध:। (अ. सू. 22/5-7)

सप्तविधा: खलु रोगा: भवन्ति-सहगर्भजातपीडाकालप्रभावस्वभावजा:। ते तु पृथक् द्विविधा:। तत्र सहजा: शुक्रार्तवदोषान्वया: कुष्ठार्शोमेहादय: पितृजा मातृजाश्च। गर्भजा जनन्यपिचारत्कौब्जपाङ्गुल्यपैङ्गल्यकिलासादयोन्नरसजा: दौह्रदविमान- जजाश्च।जातजा: स्वापचारात्सन्तर्पणजा अपतर्पणजाश्च। पीडाकृता: क्षतभङ्ग- प्रहारक्रोधशोकभयादय: शरीरामानसाश्च। कालजा: शीतादिकृता ज्वरादयो व्यापन्नजा असंरक्षणजाश्च। प्रभावजा देवगुरुल्लङ्घनशापायर्वणादिकृता ज्वरादय: पिशाचादयश्च। स्वभावजा: क्षुत्पिपासाजरादय: कालजा अकालजाश्च। तत्र कालजा रक्षणकृता: अरक्षणजा मकालजा:। त एते समासत: पुनर्द्विविधा भवन्ति प्रत्युत्पन्नकर्मजा: पूर्वकर्मजाश्च। तत्र रोगोत्पत्ति प्रत्युत्पन्नं कर्म यदनेनैव शरीरेण दृष्टमदृष्टं चोद्दिश्याप्तोपदिष्टानां विहितानां प्रतिषिद्धानामननुष्ठानमनुष्ठानं वा। जन्मान्तरातीतेन तु पूर्वकम्। तत्तु पुनर्दैवाख्यमुक्तं च नियतानियतभेदेन प्राक्।तस्मात् दृष्टहेतव: प्रत्युत्पन्नकर्मजा:। विपरीता दैवजन्मान:। अल्पनिदाना महारुजश्चोभयात्मका:।

(अ. सू. 22/3-4)

एकदोषज-द्वंद्वज-सान्निपातिका रोगा:

द्व्युल्बणैकोल्बणै: षट् स्युर्हीनमध्यादिकैश्च षट्। समैश्चैको विकारास्ते सन्नि-पातास्त्रयोदश।

संसर्गे नव षट् तेभ्य एकवृद्ध्या समैस्त्रय:।पृथक् त्रय श्चस्तैर्वृद्धैर्व्याधय: पञ्चविंशति:।

(च. सू. 17/40-41)

धातव: उपधातवश्च

स्नायौ सिराकण्डराभ्यो दृष्टा: क्लिश्नन्ति मानवम्। स्तम्भसङ्कोचखल्लीभि-र्गन्थिस्फुरणसुप्तिभि:।

(च. सू. 28/21)

रसात् स्तन्यं ततो रक्तम् असृज: कंडरा: सिरा:।
मासात् वसा त्वचा षट्च भेदस: स्नायुसंभव:।
अथ्न: दंत: ततो मज्ज: केश ओजश्च सप्तम:।
स्तन्यक्षये स्तनयोम्लानता स्तन्यासम्भवोऽल्पता वा।।   (सु. सू. 15/16)
स्तन्यं (वृद्धं) स्तनयोरापीनत्वं मुहुर्मुहु: प्रवृत्तिं तोदं च।   (सु. सू. 15/21)

मला:

मलानाश्रित्य कुपिता भेदशोषप्रदूषणम्।
दोषा मलानां कुर्वन्ति सङ्घोत्सर्गावतीव च।   (च. सू. 28/22)
कफपित्तमल: खेषु प्रस्वेदो नखरोमच।

                    (रोगविज्ञान विकृति विज्ञान–रानडे, पृ. 33–34)

रोगमार्गा:

त्रयोरोगमार्गा इति–शाखा मर्मास्थिसन्धय: कोष्ठश्च।
तत्र शाखा रक्तादयो धातवस्त्वक् च, स बाह्यो रोगामार्ग:।
    मर्माणि पुनर्बस्तिहृदयमूर्धादीनी, अस्थिसन्धयोऽस्थिसंयोगस्तत्रोपनिबद्धाश्च
स्नायुकण्डरा: स मध्यमो रोगमार्ग:।
    कोष्ठ: पुनरुच्यते–महास्रोत: शरीरमध्यं महानिम्नमामपक्वाशयश्चेति
पर्यायशब्दैस्तन्त्रे, स रोगामार्ग आभ्यन्तर:।
    तत्र गण्डपिडकालज्यचीचर्मकीलाधिमांसमषककुष्ठव्यङ्गादयो विकारा
बहिर्मार्गजाश्च विसर्पश्वयथुगुल्मार्शोविद्रध्यादय: शाखानुसारिणो भवन्ति रोगा:।
    पक्षवधग्रहापतानकार्दितशोषराजयक्ष्मास्थिसन्धिशूलगुदभ्रंशादय: शिरोह-
द्वस्तिरोगादश्च मध्यममार्गानुसारिणो भवन्ति रोगा:।
    ज्वरातीसारच्छर्द्यलसकविसूचिकाकासश्वासहिक्कानाहोदरप्लीहादयोऽन्तर्मार्गजाश्च
विसर्पश्वयथुगुल्मार्शोविद्रध्यादय: कोष्ठानुसारिणो भवन्ति रोगा:।

                                        (च. सू. 11/ 48–49)

प्रकृति–सम समवाय

विकृति–विषम–समवाय

प्रकृतिसमसमवायारब्धे तु वातजादिज्वरलिङ्गान्येव समस्तानि कतिपयानि वा भवन्ति।
अत एव चिकित्सिते चरको विकृति विषमसमवायारब्धानां द्वन्द्वसन्निपातज्वराणां
लक्षणानि साक्षात् पठित्वा निदानस्थानोक्तं वातादिज्वरलिङ्गातिदेशेन प्रवृतिसम।
समवेतानाद्वन्द्वसन्निपातज्वराणां लक्षणमुक्तवान्। यदाह– ''निदाने त्रिविधा प्रोक्ता
या पृथङ्ज्वराकृति:। संसर्गसन्निपातानां तथा चोक्तं स्वलक्षणम्'' इति।।

                                        (च. चि. 3/110, मा. नि. ज्वर 14)

एवं वक्ष्यमाणं द्वन्द्वसन्निपातलक्षणं व्याख्येयम्।प्रकृतिसमसम- वायुविकृति-
विषमसमवाययोश्चायमर्थ:-प्रकृत्या हेतुभूतया सम: कारणानुरूप: समवाय: कार्य-
कारणभावसम्बन्ध: प्रकृतिसमसमवाय:, कारणानुरूपं कार्यमित्यर्थ:, यथा-शुक्लतन्तु-
समवायारब्धस्य पटस्य शुक्लत्वम्। विकृत्या हेतुभूतया विषम: कारणानुरूप: समवायो
विकृतिविषमसमवाय:, यथा-हरिद्राचूर्णसंयोगे लौहित्यमिति।

(मा. नि. ज्वर 14)

अनुबन्ध्य-अनुबन्धी-दोषा: रोगाश्च

द्विविधा: रोगा:

ते च रोगा: सवप्रधाना भवन्त्यन्यपरिवारावाकमादननुबन्ध्यानुबन्धाया।। तत्रद्धा:
स्वतन्त्रा: स्पष्टाकृतयो तथास्वं समुत्थानोपशयाश्च इतरे तु तद्विपरीता:। तद्वच्च
दोषा: अपि। (अ. सं.
सू. 22)

तमक: कफकासेतु स्याश्चेत् पित्तानुबन्धजा:।
पित्तकासक्रिया तत्र यथावस्थं प्रयोजयेत्।।

पित्तकासे तु सकफे वमनं। पित्तकासे तनुकफे त्रिवृतां मधुरैर्हिताम्।
युञ्जयाद्रिरेकाय, युता घनश्लेष्मणि तिक्तकै:।। (अ. हृ. चि. 3/25-26)

2

AETIOLOGICAL FACTORS
(ROGANAM KARANANI)

It is the aetiological factors which increase, decrease or vitiate the various *doshas*, *dhatus* and *malas*, which in turn gives rise to various diseases.

CLASSIFICATION OF AETIOLOIRICAL FACTORS

They can be classified in various ways :

(i) *Sannikrishta and Viprakrishta*

(ii) *Pradhanika and Vyabhichari*

(iii) *Bahyahetu and Antarhetu*

(i) *Sannikrishta and Viprakrishta* : Factors like day, night, season, diet, etc. which increase *doshas* immediately are known as *sannikrishta* causes, e.g. aggravation of *asthma* at night or in spring season or on exposure to dust. In short, they are the direct and immediate cause.

When the causative factor acts indirectly after a long period, it is known as *viprakrishta*, e.g. *Kapha* keeps on accumulating in winter and disease manifests in spring. In this case, winter acts as *viprakrishta* or indirect cause while spring acts as a *sannikrishta* cause. In sort, these are remote causes.

(ii) *Pradhanika and Vyabhichari* : The most important causative factor is known as *pradhana* or *pradhanika* cause, e.g. in poisoning, poison acts as a *pradhanika* cause. The causative factor is so mild that by itself it never rise to manifest disease. The subclinical forms of the diseases are caused by *vyabhichari* factors.

(iii) *Bahyahetu and Antarhetu* : *Bahyahetu*, i.e. external causes. Enviromental factors like diet, activity, etc. can give rise to disease, if it causes in increase or decrease of *dhatus* (tissues), *doshas* or *malas* depending on whether their qualites are similar or opposite to the *dhatus, doshas* or *malas*. These waste products, i.e. *malas* accumulate by suppression of natural urges, obstruction to their passage and decrease or increased quantity of products.

Aetiological factors giving rise to various diseases are as follows :

(1) Chromosomal and genetic factors (*Bijabhagavayava-dushti*)

(2) Constitutional factors (*Doshaprakriti*)

(3) Causes of Increased *doshas* (*Doshavriddhikaranani*)

(4) Congenital anomalies (*Janmabalapravritta vikriti*)

(5) Not following dictates of one's own conscience (*Praj-naparadha*)

(6) Environmental factors, i.e. time and season (*Kalakrita*)

(7) Age (*Vaya*)

(8) Sex (*Lingabheda*)

(9) Regional factors (*Deshakrita*)

(10) Occupational factors (*Vyavasayika*)

(11) Excessive, inadequate or abnormal use of sense and motor organs (*Indri yanam hina-mithya-atiyoga*)

(12) Suppression of natural urges (*Vegavarodha*)

(13) Vitiation of body channels (*Srotodushti*)

(14) Digestive powers and tissue enzymes (*Agni*)

(15) Motility of intestines (*Koshtha*)

(16) Diet (*Ahara*)

(17) Toxins (*Ama*)

(18) Psychological factors (*Manasika*)

(19) Infectious and parasitic diseases (*Krimiroga*)

(20) Natural calamities and epidemics (*Janapadodhvansa*)

(21) Supernatural powers (*Grahabadha*)

(22) Iatrogenic factors (*Vaidyakrita*)

(23) Idiopathic or unknown factors (*Purvajanmakrita*)

(1) *Chromosomal and Genetic Factors* (*Bijabhagavayava Dushti*) : The word *Bija* means 'seed', i.e. fertilised ovum, *Bijabhaga* means chromosome, which is dervied from *bhaga* meaning, part *bija* meaning fertilised ovum. The word *bija bhagavayava* means gene which is *avayava,* i.e. part of the *bijabhaga,* i.e. chromosome.

Bijabhaga, i. e. chromosomes constitute the parts of ovum and sperm and are responsible for the hereditary characters. A defective chromosome or a part of chromosome, i.e. gene is responsible for abnormalities of sex organs and defect in a particular organ. Members of certain families are inherently predisposed to develop diabetes mellitus, recurrent attacks of common colds, asthma, etc.

Health as well as disease are primarily determined by quality of the genes. A person with all the genes of good quality leads a healthy and vigorous life of hundred years, provided he gets good food, pure air, clean water and follows the dictates of his conscience.

Genes play an important role in the causation of all natural diseases. Even in cases of infectious diseases which are caused by germs, genes determine the resistance of the tissues or organs to the infective agent, e. g. individuals born with weak respiratory tract are susceptible to frequent attacks of cold, cough or asthma. Hence, some persons hardly ever suffer from cold, while others develop cold, even on exposure to fan or after headbath.

(2) *Constitutional Factors* (*Doshaprakriti*) : Physcial and psychological constitutions are partly genetic or hereditary and partly acquired being modified by intra-uterine and extra-uterine enviromental factors as well as the diet and activities of the individual.

Amongst all constitutions, *samaprakriti*, i.e. well balanced constitution is the healthiest one. Strictly speaking persons with *Vata*, *Pitta* and *Kapha* constitution are apparently healthy. Majority of people belong to the category of diseased constitution.

These individual constitutions arc predisposed to disease by various environmental seasonal, dietary factors and activities, e.g. a person with *Vata* constitution living in *jangala*, i.e. arid region, consuming diet increasing *Vata dosha* like *chana vatana wal*, etc. and engaged in over-exertion, fasting, etc. is likely to develop *Vataja* disease. On the other hand, a person with *Vata* constitution who stays in warm and humid climate, cats diet dominant in milk, ghee, oil, meat and takes adequate rest and sleep during the day is likely to remain free from *Vataja* diseases.

A person with *Kapha* constitution is likely to develop cough, breathlessness, etc. and a person with *Pitta* constitution is likely to suffer from peptic ulcer, high fever, bleeding disorders, etc. Thus, people with *Vata*, *Pitta*, and *Kapha* constitution get off the balance easily when they are exposed to environmental and dietary factors and activities increasing that particular *dosha* and present with various clinical manifestations depending on the *dosha* affected. On the other hand, person with *sama* constitution can tolerate environmental and dietary changes and activities easily, subdue the vitiated *doshas* if any.

Health is not mere absence of any disease, but the sense of well being and joy which is usually found with those having *sama* constitution. Hence, the aim of' all individuals should be to attain balanced constitution a maintain it. As a simple and effective measure *Vata*, *Pitta* and *Kapha* constitution should take *tila* oil, ghee and honey respectively.

(3) *Factors which Increase various Doshas (Dosha Vriddhi Karanani)* : Various factors like diet, activities, environmental and psychological factors, medicines, age, etc. affect the *doshas*. These are enumerated in the following table. For details the reader may refer to pages 131-142 of my book Basic Principles of Ayurveda.

Particulars	*Vata*	*Pitta*	*Kapha*
• Environment	Cold, Dry, breeze, Storm, Cloudy weather, Cold climate	Heat, Dust, smoke, hot and dry climate	Rain, Cold and humid climate
Season	*Grishma, Varsha,* i.e. summer and rainy seasons	*Varsha, Sharad Grishma,* i.e. summer, autumn and rainy seasons	*Hemant, Shishir vasant,* i.e. spring and winter
Time of day	Evening 2 p.m. to 6 p.m.	Afternoon 10 a.m. to 2 p.m.	Morning 6 a.m. to 10 a.m.
Time of night	Late night 2 a.m. to 6 a.m.	Mid-night 10 a.m. to 2 a.m.	Early night 6 p.m. to 10 p.m.
Relation to meals	After food is completely digested	During digestion	Immediately after meals
• Diet			
Pulses	*Chana, mung. Masur, Tur, Harenu Vatana,* Beans	*Kulattha, Mustard, Udid, Atasi, Vatana*	*Udid,* Seasame seed (*Tila*)
Cereals	*Vari, Ragi, Koradush*		*Yava,* wheat, *Krishara, Prithuka* (*Poha*), *Shashkuli* (*Karanji*)
Leafy Vegetables	*Chuka,* Dry leafy vegetables	*Shringa, Velika Shaka*	Mrunal, *Bisa,* Lotus-stalk
Other Vegetables	Onion, Carrot	Drumstick, Elephant foot	*Kasheruka, Shringataka*
Fruits	*Jamun, tinduka* Watermelon	Sour fruit, *Pilu, Amrataka, Jambir*	Dates, Coconut *Mocha,* Sugarcane
Fat and Olis		*Tila* oil	Ghee
Meat		*Godha,* Fish, Goat, Sheep	Meat and fat of animals from wet region
Milk and milk products		Curds, Butter-Milk *Kurchika,* Water over curds	Milk, Curd, *Payasam,* Ghee, *Apupa, Amakshira, Kilata, Morata, Kurchika, Piyusha*
Alcohols and wines	Some types of wine		Most of the wines and alcohol
Miscellaneous	Inadequate food, Dry, food, *Kanji*	Cow's urine, *Bhallataka,* pepper *Langalika*	Preparations of sugarcane juice, Jagggery, *Phanita.*

Particulars	Vata	Pitta	Kapha
General dietetic principles	Light diet, Fasting, irregular diet, Inadequate diet	Fasting, Penance, Incompatible, diet, Indigestion, Burnt food	Indulging in tasty food, Drinking excessive amounts of water in general and at night, Eating excess of nourishing dict, Indigestion
● Panchakarma	Following excessive use of *panchakarma*		
● Natural urges	Suppression or induction of natural urges		
● Psychological factors	Fear, sorrow, eagerness, anger, worry, Study, trouble excessive joy	Anger, Fear, Sorrow, Envy	Laziness, Excessive joy
● Qualities			
Taste	Astringent, bitter and pungent.	Sour, Salty and Pungent	Sweet, sour and salty
Virya	Cold	Hot	Cold
Qualities	Dry, light, clean and Constipating food	Hot, light and fermenting food	Semisolid, oily, heavy, moist, soft, bulky, smooth and slimy food
● Activity			
Activity	Excessive activity	Excessive activity	Less activity
Exercise	Excessive + Injury, swimming carrying heavy loads travelling, controlling bullocks horses and elephants, adventures wrestling	Excessive + Exposure to sun	Lack of exercise, lazines, inactivity of body, mind and speech Rest in excess Sleeping during day Sleeping after meals
Speech	Loud and excessive	Excessive	Less
Sex	Excessive	Excessive	Less
sleep	Less, keeping awake at night	Less	Excessive sleeping during day also
● Age	Old age	Youth	Childhood

(4) *Prajnaparadha* : Not of following dictates of one's own conscience is the root cause of the illness. One often follows a wrong path inspite of knowing its consequences. Even an intelligent man falls a prey to various desires and instincts. Then what to talk about those less intelligent people, who can distinguish between the right and the wrong, the good and the bad, or those who have defective memory. The following are some of examples of *Prajnaparadha* :

   (i) Suppressing natural urges

  (ii) Undertaking unusual adventures

 (iii) Excessive indulgence in sex

 (iv) Rude behaviour

  (v) Not respecting elderly people and teachers

 (vi) Indulging in cultivated tastes rather than following natural desires and aversions

 (vii) Excessive indulgence in alcohol or other intoxicating items

(viii) Not following righteous path

 (ix) Becoming angry, jealous, frightful and greedy and acting accordingly

Lack of control over one's desires and actions, not following the dictates of one's own conscience and excessive indulgence in the worldly pleasures and non-religious acts are responsible for the decrease in life span as well as gradual decrease in health, vigour and resistance to diseases over ages, i.e. through *Krita*, *Treta*, *Dvapara* and *Kaliyugas*.

(5) *Environmental Factors (Kalakrita Karanarni)* : Life and health depend on the continuous interaction between man and his environment. The environment is never steady and keeps on changing every moment, e.g. temperature, humidity, light, sound, breeze, etc. at any place keep on fluctuating from moment to moment, morning to evening and season to season.

In summer, the dry air which we breathe in continuously and with which the skin is in constant contact would increase the dryness of the body. This in turn would result in increase of *Vata dosha* in the body which also is dry. The burning heat of october, i.e. *sharad* season would tend to increase the heat in the body, which in turn would result in increase of *Pitta dosha*, which is also hot in nature. The cold atmosphere of the winter would tend to lower the body temperature, which in turn would result in increase of *Kapha* in the body, which is cold in nature.

Time and Season : Time is eternal and exerts its effects on every living creature as well as on inanimate objects. Thus, every living creature after birth, grows, matures, degenerates (old age) and dies in course of time. Time is further divided into morning, afternoon, evening and night, various seasons, time in relation to feed.

Following table summarises the effect of time factor on the three *doshas*.

Time when a particular dosha is dominant	Vata	Pitta	Kapha
• Seasons			
Grishma	Chaya		Prashama
Vasant			Prakopa
Varsha	Prakopa	Chaya	
Sharad	Prashama	Prakopa	
Hemant		Prashama	
Shishir			Chaya
• Time of day/night	2 p.m. to 6 p.m. evening	10 a.m. to 2 p.m. afternoon	6 a.m. to10 a.m. morning
	2 a.m. to 6 p.m. late night	10 a.m. to 2 a.m. mid night	6 a.m. to early night
• Relation to food	After digestion is over	During digestion	Immediately after food intake
• Age	Old Age	Youth	Child hood

Some diseases like malaria manifest in a periodical manner. Asthmatic attacks usually occur at night. Chronic diseases like eczema, *asthma*, nephirotic syndrome tend to have seasonal aggravation. Old age and death represent natural disease, which no body can avoid.

Doshas and Season : *Vata, Pitta* and *Kapha* are naturally increased in *Varsha*, i.e. monsoon, *sharad*, i.e. autumn and *vasanta*, i.e. spring respectively. This natural increase is termed as *prakritadushti* (natural vitiation). On the other hand, if *Pitta* is increased in winter and *Kapha* is increased in summer, it is termed as *vikritadushti*, i.e. unnatural vitiation of *dosha*. Diseases arising as result of *prakritisushti* are easily cured, while those arising as a result of *vikritadushti* are difficult to cure.

(6) Age (Aayu) : Everyone passes through the stages of childhood, youth and old age marked by growth, maturity and senescence. *Kapha, Pitta* and *Vata* are the dominant *doshas* in childhood, the middle age and the closing years of life respectively Hence, *Kaphaja, Pittaja* and *Vataja* diseases are common in children, youth and old people respectively. Children have delicate tissues and organs poor resistance to infection and are likely to suffer from disorders of growth and development and *Kaphaja* diseases. Adults are prone to *Pittaja* disease like hyperacidity. Old persons are prone to *Vataja* diseases, which include various degenerative disorders and they undergo gradual loss of functions of various organs.

(7) Sex (Lingam) : The morbidity mortality in most of the diseases is generally less in females as compared to males. This may be partly explained on the basis of intermittent natural purification of the body during menstrual period. In addition, the regenerative ability of all the tissue is increased during pregnancy and lactation.

All the body channels in the females are wider and more distensible. Hence, obstructive diseases of various body channels including blood vessels, lymphatics, etc. are less common in females. Hence, coronary thrombosis, hemiplegia, etc. are less common in females.

(8) *Regional Factors (Daishika Karanani)* : Certain disease are peculiar to and are found only in certain regions. The region is classified as *anupa,* i.e. wet land, *jangala,* i.e. dry land and *sadharana*, i.e. average land.

Anupa pradesh, i.e. wet land is characterised by heavy rainfall, dense forest, marshy places and scanty breeze. The local inhabitants tend more towards *Kapha* constitution and are prone to develop *Kaphaja* diseases, i.e. diseases caused by dominance of *Kapha*.

Jangala pradesh, i.e. dry or and land has minimum or no rain fall with dry winds blowing off and on. The local inhabitants, hence tend more towards *Vata* constitution and are prone to develop *Vataja* diseases.

It is important to know the place of birth of the patient as well as the place, where he had spent his childhood and the places of origin of the disease.

(9) *Occupational Factors (Vyavasayika Karanani)* : Persons following certain profession and businessmen are more prone to develop certain diseases because of the nature of their duties, i.e. priests usually ignore their natural urges as they are busy with religious rituals. Royal attendants work under psychological tensions. Businessmen lack exercise because of the sedentary nature of their work. Prostitutes are prone to develop veneral diseases.

(10) *Excessive, Indequate or Abnormal Use of Sense and Motor Organs (Indriyanam Hina, Mithya Atiyoga)* : Normally, the interaction between various sense organs and the environmental objects, which stimulate them is well balanced. If not, body tends to attenuate or avoid it.

The following tables gives the examples of excessive, less and abnormal interaction of various sense organs and their objects

all of which give rise to diseases of that particular sense organ
and later a generalised disease.

Sense organs and senses objects	Interactions		
	Excessive	*Less*	*Abnormal*
● Hearing and sound	Hearing loud sound or hearing continuously	Not learing at all or hearing too infrequently	Hearing, harsh firghtening, impolite, unpleasant, news suggestive of impending calamities
● Skin and touch	Continuous or excessive stimulation of skin	Too less or not stimulating skin at all	Contact with poisonous substances, insects, germs and breeze; oil massage during indigestion
● Eye and light	Looking at very objects or microscopic objects	Not seeing at all	Looking at fierce, frightful or unpleasant object, looking at very near or far away object
● Nose and smell	Smelling very strong odour	Not using sense of smell at all	Smelling putrefied foul smelling, unpleasant or fermented smells
● Tongue and taste	Eating in excess tasty items	Not eating any tasty food items	Eating excess or oily, pungent, hot, sour or

Body Response (Karma) : The body response is divided
into activities of body, speech and mind. Excessive body activity
includes strenuous exercise, swimming, carrying very heavy load,
etc. Inactivity includes lying down in bed, etc. Abnormal activity
include wrestling, adventures, lying in abnormal posture, etc.
Excessive speech include singing and speaking for hours, less
speech includes observing silence and abnormal speech includes
abuses, shouting loudly, screaming, etc. Excessive activity of
mind includes studying late at night, less activity of mind includes
excessive sleep and abnormal activity includes jealousy, anger,

fear, stealing, violence, etc. Excessive physical activity would result in an increase of body heat and loss of body fluids in the form of sweating, water vapour in the exhaled air, etc. This would result in decrease of *Kapha dosha* and increase of *Vata* and *Pitta dosha* in the body. On the other hand, inactivity or excess of sleep would result in increase of *Kapha dosha.*

Psychological factors like fear and anger which result in stress and sympathetic activity increases *Vata* and *Pitta doshas* in the body. On the other hand, joy or happiness which increase para-sympathetic activity would result in increase in the *Kapha doshas* in the body.

(11) *Suppression of Natural Urges (Vegavarodha)* : *(See* chapter 4).

(12) *Vitiation of Body Channels (Srotodushti)* : *(See* chapter 5).

(13) *Enzymes (Agni)* : *(See* chapter 6).

(14) *Motility of Intestines (Koshtha)* : Depending on the peristalic movements a person's bowel may by classified as a hyperactive bowel, i.e. *mridu koshtha,* medium bowel, i.e. *madhyamakoshtha* and sluggish bowel, i.e. *krura koshtha.* A person with hyperactive bowel may start purging by taking two cups of milk, eating grapes or drinking wine. One the other hand, a purgative hardly ever acts in a person with sluggish bowel, i.e. *krura koshtha.* Dominance of *Vata dosha* leads to sluggish bowel, i.e. *krura koshtha,* while dominance of *Pitta dosha* leads to hyper-active bowel, i.e. *mridu koshtha.* Persons with sluggish bowel are usually constipated, while persons with hyperactive bowel tend to have loose stools. In a person with sluggish bowel, one has to administer oil and ghee for seven days for adequate oleation of bowel, i.e. *samyak snehana.* On the other hand, three days are enough for adequate oleation in a person with hyperactive bowel.

A person with balance activity of bowel is termed as having *sama koshtha.* Person with *madhya koshtha* will develop consti-pation or diarrhoea on administration of diet like milk or leafy vegetables respectively. On the other hand, a person with *sama koshtha* will tolerate both types of food without developing constipation or diarrhoea.

(15) **Dietetic Factor (Aharaja)** : *(See* chapter 7*).*

(16) **Toxins (Ama)** : *(See* chapter 8*).*

(17) **Pshchological Causes (Manasika Karanami)** : Psycological like tension, fear and anger are responsible for psychic diseases like insanity, *atatvabhinivesha,* epilepsy, etc. psychological causes also lead to diseases of body like diarrhoea, heart diseases, diseases of body channels, etc. by vitiating *Vata, Pitta* or *Kapha.*

(18) **Infectious and Parasitic Diseases (Krimiroga)** : *(See* chapter 9*).*

(19) **Natural Calamities and Epidemics (Janapadodhvansa)** : *(See* chapter 10*).*

(20) **Supernatural Powers (Grahabadha)** : *(See* chapter 11*).*

(21) **Iatrogenic Diseases (Vaidyakrita)** : If the physician or the nurse commits any mistake while prescribing or administering the treatment, it may lead to unexpected or more severe form of ailment or complication, which is termed as iatrogenic disease. Excessive, less or wrong use of any therapeutic measure may lead to iatrogenic disease.

(22) **Unknown Factors (Karanani Praktana)** : The aetological or causative factors of the disease can be divided into (i) Known factors, and (ii) Unknown factors, where it is not possible to demonstarate realation between cause and effect. The known causes are either environmental factors or *prajnyaparadha,* i.e. not following dictates of one's own conscience as we have seen before. Some of the unknown cause can be explained on the basis of hereditary or constitutional weakness, However, why should only a particular child of the same parents suffer from hereditary disease or constitutional flaws. At present, the physicians put these unknown factors as fate, destiny, nature, bad luck, etc.

Indian philosophers believe that these unknown factors are the fruits of sins of past lives as well as of present life maturing in this very life. Neither God nor the demons or ghosts torment man. Man himself is responsible for the painful or comfortable state of his health.

रोगाणाम् कारणानि

सन्निकृष्ठ-विप्रकृष्ट कारणानि

सन्निकृष्टविप्रकृष्टव्यभिचारिप्रधानिकभेदाच्चतुर्धा इति। सन्निकृष्टो यथा-नक्तंदिनर्तुभुक्तांशा दोषप्रकोपस्य हेतव:, न ते चयादिकमपेक्षन्ते। विप्रकृष्टे यथा-''हेमन्ते निचित: श्लेष्मावसन्ते कफरोगकृत्''; किंवा सन्निकृष्टोज्वरस्य रुक्षादिसेवा विप्रकृष्टे रुद्रकोप:।

व्यभिचारी- प्रधानिक कारणानि

यथा-यो दुर्बलत्वाद्व्याधिकरणासमर्थ:। यदाह चरक:, '' (निदानादि विशेषा) अबलीयांसोऽथवानुबन्धन्ति न तदा विकाराभिनिवृत्ति:'' इति।

(च. नि. स्था. -4)

प्राधानिको यथा-विषादि:।

(मा. नि. 5 टीका पृ. 7-8)

व्याभिचारी- इह खलु निदानदोषदूष्येभ्यो विकारविधातभावाभावप्रतिविशेषा भवन्ति। यदा ह्येते त्रयो निदानादिविशेषा: परस्परं नानुबध्नन्त्यथवा कालप्रकर्षादब-लीयांसोऽथवाऽनुबन्धन्ति न तदा विकाराभिनिर्वृत्ति:।

(च. नि. 4/4)

व्यावसायिक रोगा:

वृत्युपायान्निषेवेत ये स्युर्धर्माविरोधिन:।

(च. सू. 5/104)

सदाऽऽतुरा: श्रोत्रियराजसेवकास्तथैव वेश्या वह पण्यजीविभि:।

(च. सि. 11/27)

द्विजो हि वेदाध्ययनव्रताह्निककृयादिभिर्देहहितं न चेष्टते।
नृपोपसेवी नृपचित्तरक्षणाद् परानुरोधाद् बहुचिन्तनाद् भयात्।
नृचित्तवर्तिन्युपचारतत्परा मृजाविभूषानिरता पणाङ्गना।
सदासनादत्यनुबन्धविक्रयक्रयादिलोभादपि पण्यजीविन:।। सदैव ते ह्यागतवेगनिग्रहं समाचरन्ते न च कालभोजनम्।
अकालनिहारविहारसेविनो भवन्ति येऽन्येऽपि सदाऽऽतुराश्च ते।

(च. सि. 11/28-30; रो. वि.वि. वि. पृ. 168, 169)

बीजभागदोषज रोगा:

सन्ति खल्वस्मिन् गर्भे केचिन्नित्या भावा:, सन्ति चानित्या: केचित्। तस्य य एवाङ्गावयवा: सन्तिष्ठन्ते, त एव स्त्रीलिङ्गं पुरुषलिङ्गं नपुंसकलिङ्गं वा बिभ्रति। तत्र स्त्रीपुरुषयोर्ये वैशेषिका भावा: प्रधानसंश्रया गुणसंश्रयाश्च, तेषां यतो भूयस्त्वं ततोऽन्य- तरभाव:।   (च. शा. 4/14)

तद्यथा–क्लैब्यं भीरुत्वमवैशारद्यं मोहोऽनवस्थानमधोगुरुत्वमसहनं शैथिल्यं मार्दवं गर्भाशयबीजभागस्तथायुक्तानि चापराणि स्त्रीकराणि, अतो विपरीतानि पुरुषकराणि, उभयभागावयवा नपुंसककराणि भवन्ति।   (च. शा. 4/14)

यदा स्त्रिया दोषप्रकोपणोक्तान्यासेवमानाया दोषा: प्रकुपिता: शरीरमुपसर्पन्त: शोणितगर्भाशयावुपपद्यन्ते, न च कार्त्स्न्येन शोणितगर्भाशयौ दूषयन्ति, तदेयं गर्भं लभते स्त्री; तदा यस्य गर्भस्य मातृजानामवयवानामन्यतमोऽवयवो विकृतिमापद्यत एकोऽथवाऽनेके,यस्य यस्य ह्यवयवस्य बीजे बीजभागे वा दोषा: प्रकोपमापद्यन्ते, तं तमवयवं विकृतिराविशति।

यदा ह्यास्या: शोणिते गर्भाशयबीजभाग: प्रदोषमापद्यते, तदा वन्ध्यां जनयति; यदा पुनरस्या: शोणिते गर्भाशयबीजभागावयव: प्रदोषमापद्यते, तदा पूतिप्रजां जनयति; यदा त्वस्या: शोषिते गर्भाशयबीजभागावयव: स्त्रीकारणां च शरीरबीजभागानामेकदेश: प्रदोषमापद्यते, तदा स्त्र्यकृतिभूयिष्ठामस्त्रियं वार्तां नाम जनयति, तां स्त्रीव्या- पदमाचक्षते।   (च. शा. 4/30)

बीजभागावयवज रोगा:

एवमेव पुरुषस्य यदा बीजे बीजभाग: प्रदोषमापद्यते, तदा वन्ध्यं जनयति; यदा पुनरस्य बीजे बीजभागावयव: प्रदोषमापद्यते तदा पूतिप्रजं जनयति; यदात्वस्य बीजे बीजभागावयव: पुरुषकरणां च शरीरबीजभागानामेकदोष: प्रदोषमापद्यते, तदा पुरुषाकृतिभूयिष्ठमपुरुषं तृणपुत्रिकं नाम जनयति; तां पुरुषव्यापदमाचक्षते।

                                                         (च. शा. 4/31)

शरीरदोषा: मानसिक दोषाश्च

तत्र त्रय: शरीरदोषा वातपित्तश्लेष्माण:, ते शरीरं दूषयन्ति; द्वौ पुन: सत्त्वदोषौ रजस्तमश्च, तौसत्त्वं दूषयत:। ताभ्यां च सत्त्वशरीराभ्यां दुष्टाभ्यां विकृतिरूपजायते, नोपजायते चाप्रदुष्टाभ्याम्।   (च. शा. 4/34)

हृद्धिविमानने दोषा:

मातृजं चास्य हृदयं मातृहृदयेनाभिसम्बद्धं भवति रसवाहिनीभि: संवाहिनीभि:, तस्मात्

तयोस्ताभिर्भक्ति: संस्पन्दते। तच्चैव कारणमवेक्षमाणा न द्वैह्रदय्यस्य विमानितं गर्भमिच्छन्ति कर्तुम्।

विमानने ह्रास्य दृश्यते विनाशो विकृतिर्वा समानयोगक्षेमा हि तदा भवति गर्भेण केषुचिदर्थेषु माता। तस्मात् प्रियहिताभ्यां गर्भिणीं विशेषेणोपचरिन्त कुशला:।

(च. शा. 4/5)

प्रार्थनासंधारणेदोषा:

तीव्रायां तु खलु प्रार्थनायां काममहितमप्यस्यै हितेनोपहितं दद्यात् प्रार्थनाविनयनार्थम्। प्रार्थनासन्धारणाद्धि वायु: प्रकुपितोऽन्त:शरीरमनुचरन् गर्भस्यापद्यमानस्य विनाशं वैरूप्यं वा कुर्यात्।

(च. शा. 4/19)

इमांश्चान्यानुपदिशन्ति वृद्धा:–देवतारक्षोऽनुचरपरिरक्षणार्थं न रक्तानि वासांसि बिभृयान् मदकराणि मद्यान्यभ्यवहरेन् यानमधिरोहेन् मांसमश्नीयात् सर्वेन्द्रियप्रतिकूलांश्च भावान् दूरत: परिवर्जयेत्, यच्चान्यदपि किञ्चित् स्त्रियो विदु:।

(च. शा. 4/19)

एतेन मातृजानां पितृजानां चावयवानां विकृतिव्याख्यानेन सात्म्यजानां रसजानां सत्त्वजानां चावयवानां विकृतिर्व्याख्याता भवति। (च. शा. 4/32)

वातपित्तकफदोषाणाम् क्षयोवृद्धि:

वातप्रकोपहेतव:

तत्र बलवद्विग्रह, अतिव्यायाम, अव्यायाम, अध्ययन प्रपतन, प्रधावन, प्रपीडन, अभिघात, लङ्घनप्लवन तरण, रात्रिजागरण भारहरण, गजतुरगरथपदातिचर्या, कटुकषायतिक्तरुक्षलघुशीतवीर्य शुष्कशाक, वल्लूरवरकोद्दालक कोरदूषश्यामाकनीवार मुद्गमसूरढकीहरेणुकलायनिष्पावानशनविषमाशन अध्यशन वातमूत्रपरीषशुक्रच्छर्दि– क्षवथूद्गारबाष्पवेगविधातादिभि विशेषै: वायु: प्रकोपमापद्यन्ते।

(सु. सू. 21/19)

धातुक्षयात् तथा मार्गस्यावरणेन वेगप्रतिबन्धयवायु: कुपितो भवति। (च. चि. 28/59)

रूक्षलघुशीतवमनविरेचनास्थापनशिरोविरेचन अतियोग व्यायामवेगासन्धारणानशन अभिघातव्यवाय उद्वेगशोकशोणितातिषेकजागरणविषमशरीरन्यासेभ्यो अतिसेवितेभ्यो वायु: प्रकोपमापद्यते।

(च. नि. 1/13)

उष्णेन युक्ता रूक्षाद्यावायो: कुर्वन्ति सञ्चयम्।

शीतेन कोपमुष्णेन शमं स्निग्धादयो गुणा:।।

(अ. ह. सू. 12/20)

चयप्रकोपप्रशमा वायोर्ग्रीष्मादिषु त्रिषु ।

वर्षादिषु तु पित्तस्य श्लेष्मण: शिशिरादिषु ।।

चीयते लघुरूक्षाभिषधीभि:समीरण: ।

तद्विधस्तद्विधे देहे कालस्यौष्ण्यान्न कुप्यति ।।

अद्भिरम्लविपामाभिरषधीभिश्च तादृशम् ।।   (अ. ह्र. सू. 12/21, 25–26)

तिक्तोष्णकषायरससेवनै: तथावर्षासु अहोरात्रिभुक्तान्ते च समीकरण: कुप्यति ।

                                               (अ.सं.नि. 15)

अन्यदोषपूर्णेभ्य: स्रोतोभ्य: आवरणं प्राप्त बलीवान: कुप्यति ।   (अ. सं. नि. 15)

तिक्तोषणकषायाल्परूक्षप्रमितभोजनै: ।

धारणोदीरणनिशाजागरतुच्चभाषणै: ।।

क्रियातियोगभिशोकचिन्ताव्यायाममैथुनै: ।

ग्रीष्माहोरात्रि भुक्तान्ते प्रकुप्यति समीरण: ।।   (अ. ह्र. नि. 1/14–15)

वातक्षयहेतव:

वातगुणस्यविपरीतगुणानां स्निग्धगुरूष्णादीनां देहे वर्धनेनवातदोषस्य क्षयो भविति ।

                                                      (अ. ह्र. सू. 11/24)

गुरुस्निधदिभिरोषधीभि: वातस्यशमोभवति ।   (अ. ह्र. सू. 12/24)

उष्णेनाशमं स्निग्धदयो गुणा: ।   (अ. ह्र. सू. 12/15)

पित्तप्रकोपहेतव:

शीतेन युक्तातीक्ष्णाद्याश्चयं पित्तस्य कुर्वते ।

उष्णेनं कोपं मन्दाद्या: शमं शीतोपसंहिता: ।।   (अ. ह्र. सू. 12/20)

चयप्रकोपप्रशमा वायो: ग्रीष्मादिषु त्रिषु ।

वर्षादिषु तु पित्तस्य श्लेष्मण: शिशिरादिषु ।।   (अ. ह्र. सू. 12/20)

अद्भिरम्लविपाकाभिषधीभिश्च तादृशम् ।।

पित्तं याति चयं कोपं न तु कालस्य शैत्यत: ।   (वा. सू. 12/26)

पित्तं कट्वम्लतीक्ष्णोष्णपटुक्रोध विदाहिभि: ।

शरन्मध्याह्राद्रात्र्यर्धविदाहसमयेषु च ।

उष्णाम्लवणक्षारकटुकाजीर्ण भोजनेभ्योऽतिसेवितेभ्यरतथा तीक्ष्णातपाग्निसन्ताप श्रमक्रोधविषमाहारेभ्यश्च पित्तं-कोपमापद्यते ।

                                                         (च. नि. 1/22)

कफप्रकोपहेतव:

क्रोधशोकभयायासोपवास विदग्धमैथुनोपगमन, कट्वम्ललवणतीक्ष्णोष्ण लघुविदा-
हितिलतैल पिण्याककुलत्थ सर्वपातसी।

चयप्रकोपप्रशमा वायोर्ग्रीष्मादिषु त्रिषु।

वर्षादिषु तुपित्तस्थ, श्लेष्मण: शिशिरादिषु।।   (अ. हृ. सू. 12/24)

शीतेनयुक्ता: स्निग्धाद्या: कुर्वते श्लेष्मणश्चयम्।

उष्णेन कोपं, तेनैव गुणा रुक्षाय:।।   (अ. हृ. सू. 12/21)

स्निग्धगुरुमधुरपिच्छिलशीताम्ललवणशममृदिवास्वप्नसहर्षव्यायामेभ्योऽतिसेवितेभ्य:
श्लेष्मा प्रकोपमापद्यते।   (च. नि. 12/25)

दितास्वप्नव्यायामालस्य, मधुराम्ललवणशीत, स्निग्धगुरुपिच्छिल अभिष्यन्दि
हायनकयवक नैषधइत्यकमाष महाभाषा, गोधूमतिलपिष्टिविकृति, दधि, दुग्ध, कृशय,
पायस, इक्षु विकारानूपौदकमांसवसा बिसमृणालकसेरुक शृङ्गाटक मधुरवल्ली,
फलसमशनाध्यशनप्रभृतिभि: श्लेष्मा प्रकोपमापद्यते।   (सु. सू. 21/23)

स्वाद्वम्ललवणस्निग्ध गुर्विभिष्यन्दिशीतलै:।

आस्यास्वप्नसुखाजीर्णदिवास्वप्नातिबृंहणै:।

प्रच्छर्दनाद्ययोगेन भुक्तमात्रवसन्तयो:।

पूर्वाह्णे पूर्वरात्रे च श्लेष्मा द्वन्द्व तु सङ्क्षरत्।।   (अ. हृ. नि. 1)

दोषस्य क्षय, वृद्धि प्रकोण लक्षण विषये सामान्य नियमानि

वाते पित्ते कफे चैव क्षीणे लक्षणमुच्यते।

कर्मण: प्राकृताद्धानि वृद्धिर्वाऽऽपि विरोधिनाम्।   (च. सू. 18/52)

वातक्षयलक्षणानि

तत्र वात क्षये-मन्दचेष्टताल्पवाक्तमप्रहर्षोमूढसंज्ञता।   (सु. सू. 15)

लिङ्गक्षीणेऽनिलेऽङ्गस्य सादोऽल्पं भाषिते हितम्।

संज्ञामोहस्तथा श्लेष्मवृद्ध्युक्तामयसम्भव:।।   (अ. हृ. सू. 11/15)

वातवृद्धिलक्षणानि

तत्र वातवृद्धौ-वाक्पारुष्यंकार्श्य काष्ण्र्य गात्रस्फुरणं।

उष्णकामिता निद्रानाशोऽल्पबलत्वं गाढवर्चस्त्वं च।।   (सु. सू. 13/13)

कार्श्यकाष्ण्यर्योष्णकामत्वकम्पानाहशकृद्ग्रहान्।

बलनिद्रेन्द्रियभ्रंशप्रलापभ्रमदीनता।   (अ. हृ. सू. 11/16)

वातप्रकोपलक्षणानि

स्रंसव्यासव्यधस्वापसादरुक्तोदभेदनम्।।

सङ्गाङ्गभङ्गसङ्कोच वर्तहर्षणतर्षणम्।।

कम्पपारुष्यसौषिर्यशोषस्पन्दनवेष्टनम्।।

स्तम्भ: कषायरसता वर्ण: श्यावोऽरुणोऽपि वा।   (अ. ह. 12/50)

स्वंय लिङ्गमिति कुपितस्य वायो रौक्ष्यादयो धर्मा:, कर्माणि च स्रंसशूलादिनी। यदाह चरकपाठसंवादी सुदान्तसेन।। आध्मवानस्तम्भरौक्ष्यस्फुटनविमथनजक्षोभकम्पप्रतोदा:। कण्ठध्वंसावदौ श्रमकविलापनं स्रंसशूलप्रमेदा:। पारुष्मं कर्णनादौ विषमपरिणतिभ्रंश-दृष्टिप्रमोहा, विस्पन्दनोद्घट्टानि ग्लपनमशयनं ताडनं पीडनं च। नामोन्नामौ विषादो भ्रमपापरितनं जृम्भणंरोमहर्षो, विक्षेपाक्षेपशोकशोषग्रहणशुषिरताश्छेदनं वेष्टनं च। वर्ण: श्यावोऽरुणो वा तृडपि च महती स्वापविश्लेषसङ्ग्ना। विद्यात् कर्माण्यमूनि प्रकुपितमरुत: स्यात् कषायो रसश्च।

                                       (मधुकोश टीका मा. नि. 1)

तं तं शरीरावयमाविशत:– तद्यथा स्रंस, भ्रंश, व्यासंगभेद हर्षतर्ष वर्त मर्द कम्प चालतोद्वयथा चेष्टादीनि। तथा खरपरुष विशद सुषिरतारुण कषायविरस मुखशोषशूल सुप्ति, संकुंचन स्तम्भन स्वजातादीनि च वायो: कर्माणि। तैरन्वितं तात्विकारमेवाध्य-वस्येत्।।   (च. सू. 2/11)

पित्तक्षयलक्षणानि

पित्तक्षये मन्दोष्माग्निता निष्प्रभत्वं च।।   (सु. सू. 15)

पित्ते मन्दोऽनल:शीतं प्रभाहानि:।।   (अ. ह. सू. 11/16)

पित्तवृद्धिलक्षणानि

पित्तवृद्धौ पितावभासता सन्तपा: शीतकामित्वम्, अल्पनिद्रता मूर्च्छा बलहानि: इन्द्रियदौर्बल्यं पीतविण्मूत्रनेत्रत्वं च।।   (सु. सू. 15/8)

पीतविण्मूत्रनेत्रत्वक्षुत्तृउदाहाल्पनिद्रता:।

पित्तम् ⋯⋯⋯⋯⋯⋯⋯⋯⋯⋯⋯⋯⋯⋯।   (अ. ह. सू. 11/7)

पित्तप्रकोपलक्षणानि

तं शरीरावयवमाविशत: (तद्यथा) दाहौष्ण, पाक स्वेद कण्डूस्त्रावरागा: यथा स्वं च गन्धवर्णरसाभि निर्वर्तनं श्रेष्मस्य कर्माणि।

तैरविन्तं पित्तविकारमेवाध्यवस्येत्।।   (च. सू. 20/18)

विस्फोटाम्लकधूमका: प्रलपनंस्वेदस्रुति मूर्च्छिने ।

दौर्गन्ध्यं दारागंमन्दोविसरणं पाकोsरतितृड्भ्रमौ ।।

ऊष्मातृप्तितमप्रवेश दहनं कट्वम्लतिक्तारसा ।

वर्ण: पाण्डुविवर्जित: क्वथितया कर्माणि पित्तस्य वै ।।

(मधुकोश टीका मा. नि. 5)

पित्तस्य दाहरागोष्मपाकिता: ।

स्वेद: क्लेद: स्रुति: कोथ: सदनं मूर्च्छनं मद: ।

कटुकाम्लौ रसौ वर्ण: पाण्डुरारुणवर्जित: ।।   (अ. ह. सू. 12/52)

कफक्षयलक्षणानि

श्लेष्मक्षये रूक्षतान्तर्दाह आमाशयेतरश्लेष्माशयशून्यता सन्धिशैथिल्यं तृष्णा दौर्बल्यं

प्रजागरणं च ।   (सु. सू. 15/11)

कफे भ्रम: ....

श्लेष्माशयानां शून्यत्वं हृद्द्रव: श्लथसन्धिता ।।   (अ. ह. सू. 11/16)

कफवृद्धिलक्षणानि

श्लेष्मवृद्धौ शौक्ल्यं शैत्यं स्थैर्य्य गौरवमवसादस्तन्द्रा निद्रा सन्ध्यस्थिविश्लेषश्च ।

(सु. सू. 15/13)

श्लेष्माऽग्निसदनप्रसेकालस्यगौरवम् ।

श्वैत्यशैत्यश्लथाङ्गत्वं श्वासकासातिनिद्रता: ।।   (अ. ह. सू. 11/7)

कफप्रकोपलक्षणानि

श्लेष्मण: स्नेह काठिण्य कण्डू शीतत्व गौरवम् ।

बन्धोपलेप स्तैमित्य शोफापक्ततिनिद्रता ।

वर्णश्वेतोरसौस्वादुलवणौ चिरकारिता ।।   (अ. ह. सू. 12/5)

तृप्तिस्तन्द्रागुरुता स्तैमित्यं कठिनता मलाधिक्यम् ।

स्नेहापक्त्युपलेपशैत्यं कण्डू: प्रसेकश्च ।।

चिरकर्तृत्वं शोथो निद्राधिक्यं रसौ पटस्वादु ।

वर्ण: श्वेतोऽलसता कर्माणि कफस्य जानीयात् ।   (मधुकोश टीका-मा. नि.)

तं तं शरीरावयवमाविशत्। श्वैत्यशैत्यकण्डूस्थैर्यगौरवस्नेहसुप्तिक्लेदोपदेह बन्धमाधुर्य

चिरकारित्वानि श्लेष्मण: कर्माणि, तैर्विन्तं श्लेष्मविकरमेवाध्यवसेत् ।।

(च. सू. 20/22)

प्राणप्रकोप:

वायौपश्चात्मके प्राणो रौक्ष्यव्यायामलङ्घनै:।

अत्याहाराभिघाताध्ववेगोदीरणधारणै:।।

कुपितश्चक्षुरदीनामुपघातं प्रवर्जयेत्।

पीनसार्दिततृट्कासश्वासादींश्चामयान्बहून्।।

उदानवायुप्रकोप:

उदान: क्षवथूद्गारछर्दिनिद्राविधारणै:।

गुरुभारातिरुदितहास्याद्यैविकृतो गदान्।।

कण्ठरोधमनोभ्रंशच्छर्द्यरोचकपीनसान्।

कुर्याच्च गलगण्डादींस्तांस्तान् जत्रूर्ध्वसंश्रयान्।।

व्यानप्रकोप:

व्यानोऽतिगमनध्यानक्रीडाविषमचेष्टितै:।

विरोधरूक्षभीहर्षविषादाद्यैश्च दूषित:।।

पुंस्त्वोत्साहबलभ्रंशशोकचित्तोत्प्लवज्वरान्।

सर्वाङ्गरोगनिस्तोदरोमहर्षाङ्गसुप्तता:।

कुष्ठं विसर्पमन्याश्च कुर्यात्सर्वाङ्गगान् गदान्।

समानवायुप्रकोप:

समानाविषमाजीर्ण शीतसङ्गीर्णभोजनै:।।

करोत्यकालशयनजागराद्यैश्च दूषित:।

शूलगुल्मग्रहण्यादीन् पक्वामाशयजान् गदान्।।

अपानवायुप्रकोप:

अपानोरूक्षगुर्वन्नवेगाघातातिवाहनै:।

यानयानासनस्थानचङ्क्रमैश्चातिसेवितै:।।

कुपित: कुरुते रोगान् कृच्छ्रान् पक्वाशयाश्रयान्।

मूत्रशुक्रप्रदोषार्शोगुदभ्रंशादिकान् बहून्।।　　　(अ. हृ. नि. 16/19–28)

प्रज्ञापराध:

धीधृतिस्मृतिविभ्रंश: सम्प्राप्ति: कालकर्मणाम्।

असात्म्यार्थागमश्चेति ज्ञातव्या दु:खहेतव:।।

विषमाभिनिवेषो यो नित्यानित्ये हिताहिते ।

ज्ञेय: स बुद्धिविभ्रंश: समं बुद्धिर्हि पश्यति ।।

विषयप्रवणं सत्त्वं धृतिभ्रंशान शक्यते ।

नियन्तु महितादर्थाद् धृतिर्हि नियमात्मिका ।।

तत्त्वज्ञाने स्मृतिर्यस्य रजोमोहावृतात्मन: ।

भ्रश्यते स स्मृतिभ्रंश: स्मर्तव्यं हि स्मृतौ स्थितम् ।।

धीधृतिस्मृतिविभ्रष्ट: कर्म यत् कुरुतेऽशुभम् ।।

प्रज्ञापराधं तं विद्यात् सर्वदोषप्रकोपणम् ।।

(च. शा. 1/97-98, 101-102)

सर्वेषामप्यग्निनिवेश वाय्वादीनां यद्वैगुण्यमुत्पद्यते तस्य मूलधर्म: ।

तन्मूलं वाऽसत्कर्म पूर्वकृतं; तयोर्योनि: प्रज्ञापराध एव ।।   (च. वि. 3/20)

प्रज्ञापराधात् सम्भूते व्याधौ कर्मज आत्मन: ।

नाभिसंसेद् बुधो देवान्पितृन् च राक्षसान् ।।

(च. वि. 37)

उदीरणं गतिमतामुदीर्णानां च निग्रह: ।

सेवनं साहसानां च नारीणां चातिसेवनम् ।

कर्मकालातिपातश्च मिथ्यारम्भश्च कर्मणाम् ।।

विनयाचारलोपश्च पूज्यानां चाभिघर्षणम् ।।

ज्ञातानां स्वयमर्थानामहितानां निषेवणम् ।

परमौन्मादिकानां च प्रत्ययानां निषेवणम् ।।

अकालादेशसञ्चारौ मैत्री सङ्क्लिष्टकर्मभि: ।

इन्द्रियोपक्रमोक्तस्य सद्वृत्तस्य च वर्जनम् ।।

(च. शा. 1)

ईर्ष्यामानभयक्रोधलोभमोहमदभ्रमा: ।

तज्जं वा कर्म यत् क्लिष्टं क्लिष्टं यद् देहकर्म च ।।

यच्चान्यदीदृशं कर्म रजोमोहसमुत्थितम् ।

प्रज्ञापराधं तं शिष्टा ब्रुवते व्याधिकारणम् ।।

बुद्ध्या विषमविज्ञानं विषमं च प्रवर्तनम् ।

प्रज्ञापराधं जानीयान्मनसो गोचरं हि तत् ।   (च. शा. 1/107-109)

प्रज्ञा च यदपराध्यति तदपि कृत्रेतादि कालवशेन । न हि आदिकाले पूर्वकृतमासीत् आशुभकर्मजं अशुभकर्मजं फलं किमपि ये बुद्धिपराध्येत। तदा कालविशेष एव प्रज्ञापराधे हेतु: कालो हि स्वभावत: शुभाऽशुभ हेतु: प्रासिध्दासितथ्यादि योगेनानुमेय:, तद् हेतुकजं प्राक्कर्म यदशुभं अशुभकाले समागते प्रज्ञातत्त्वविदामत्त्वविदां चापराध्यति,

तत् कालजं प्रज्ञापराधजं तत्फलमधर्म: परिणाम एवं उच्यते। आदि कारणतो हि
संज्ञा भवति फलजननं प इदानीं कालेन परिणामादेवेति परिणामे धर्माऽधर्मान्तर्भावो
न प्रज्ञापराध समयोगायोरिति।   (च. नि. 1- गंगाधर टीका)

परिणाम

निर्दिष्ट: कालसंज्ञाप्तिव्याधिसङ्ग्रहे।
चयप्रकोपप्रशमा: पित्तादीनां यथा पुरा।।
मिथ्यातिहीनलिङ्गाश्च वर्षान्ता रोगहेतव:।
जीर्णभुक्तप्रजीर्णान्नकालाकालस्थितिश्च या।।
पूर्वमध्यापराह्णाश्च रात्रा यामास्त्रयश्च ये।
एषु कालेषु नियता ये रोगास्ते च कालजा:।।
अन्येद्युष्को द्वयहग्राही तृतीयकचतुर्थकौ।
स्वे स्वे काले प्रवर्तन्ते काले द्वेषां बालगम:।।
एते चान्ये च ये केचित् कालजा विविधा गदा:।
अनागते चिकित्स्यान्ते बलकालौ विजानता।।
कालस्य परिणामेन जरामृत्युनिमित्तजा।
रोगा: स्वभाविका दृष्टा: स्वभावो निष्प्रतिक्रिय:।।
निर्दिष्टं दैवशब्देन कर्म यत् पौर्वदेहिकम्।
हेतुस्तदपि कालेन रोगाणामुपलभ्यते।।
नहि कर्म महात् किञ्चित्फलं यस्य न भुज्यते।
क्रियाध्नां कर्मजारोगा: प्रशमं यान्ति तत्क्षणात्।।   (च. शा. 10/109-116)

असात्म्य इन्द्रियार्थ संयोग

कालार्थकर्मणा योगो हीनामिथ्यातिमात्रक:।
सम्यग्योगश्च विज्ञेय: रोगारोग्यैककारणम्।।   (अ. ह. सू. 1/19)

तेषां कोपे तु कारण

अर्थैरसात्मै: संयोग: काल: कर्म च दुष्कृताम्।
हीनातिमथ्यातियोगेन भिद्यते तत्पुनस्त्रिधा।।   (अ. ह. सू. 12/35)
असात्म्यमिति तद्विद्घादयन्नयाति सहात्मताम्।   (च. शा. 1/27)
हीनोऽर्थेनेन्द्रियस्याल्प: संयोग: स्वेन नैव वा।
अतियोगोऽतिसंसर्ग:, सूक्ष्मभासुरभैरवम्।।

अत्यास्नतिदूरस्थं विप्रियं विकृतादि च।
यदक्ष्णा वीक्ष्यते रूपं मिथ्यायोग: स दारुण:।। (अ. हृ. सू. 12/36, 37)

अत्युग्रशब्दश्रवणाच्छ्रवणात् सर्वशो न च।
शब्दानां चातिहीनानां भवन्ति श्रवणाज्जडा:।।
पुरुषोद्भदीषणाशस्ताप्रियव्यसन सूचकै:।
शब्दै: श्रवणसंयोगो मिथ्यासंयोग उच्यते।।
असंस्पर्शोऽति संस्पर्शो हीनसंस्पर्श एव च।
स्पृश्यानां संग्रहेणोक्त: स्पर्शनेन्द्रियबाधक:।।
यो भूतविषवातानामकालेनागतश्च य:।
स्नेहशीतोष्णसंस्पर्शो मिथ्यायोग: स उच्यते।।
रूपाणां भास्वतां दृष्टिर्विनश्यति दर्शनात्।
दर्शनाचाति सूक्ष्माणां सर्वशश्चाप्यदर्शनात्।।
द्विष्टैर्भैरवबीभत्सदूरातिशिलष्ट दर्शनात्।
तामसानां च रूपाणां मिथ्यासंयोग उच्यते।।
अत्यादानमनादानमोकसात्याादिभिश्च यत्।
रसानां विषमादानमल्पादानं च दूषणम्।।
अतिमृद्वतितीक्ष्णानां गन्धानामुपसेवनम्।
असेवनं सर्वशश्च घ्राणेन्द्रियविनाशनम्।।
पूतिभूतविषद्विष्टा गन्धा ये चाप्यनार्तवा:।
तैर्गन्धैर्घ्राणसंयोगो मिथ्यायोग: स उच्यते।। (च. शा. 1/118–126)

कर्म

कायवाक्चित्तभेदेन कर्मापि विभजेत्रिधा।
कायादिकर्मणां हीना प्रवृत्तिर्हीनसंज्ञिका।।
अतियोगोति वृत्तिस्तुऽवेगोदीरणधारणम्।
विषमाङ्गशक्रियारम्भपतनस्खलनादिकम्।।
भाषणं सामिभुक्तस्य रागद्वेषभयादि च।
कर्मप्राणातिपातादि दशधा यच्च निन्दितम्।।
मिथ्यायोग: समस्तोऽसाविह वाऽमुत्र वा कृतम्। (अ. हृ. सू. 12/ 39–42)

3

CONGENITAL ANOMALIES
(JANMABALA PRAVRITTA VYADHI)

Ayurveda describes many congenital anomalies, i.e. *jammabalapravritta vyadhi* such as *andhya* (blindness), *badhirya* (deafness), *muka* (dumbness), *vriddhi* congenital hernia, *sanniruddha guda* (anal atresia or stenosis), *sahaja arsha* (congenital anomalies) of the sexual organs, etc.

AETIOLOGY

Congenital anomalies may be genetic in origin or may arise as a result of factors operating in the intrauterine life. Consanguintity is known to be associated with increased incidence of congenital defects. Hence, the religious texts prescribe that the prospective parents should not be related to each other and should not belong to the same family tree for seven previous generations.

The acquired factors operate on the foetus, viz. diet, activity, disease, psychological factors, etc. of the mother. They act by disturbing the balance of *doshas* in the pregnant woman and later in the foetus. The increased, decreased or vitiated *doshas* in the foetus give rise to congenital anomalies.

The various causes giving rise to congenital anomalies are given below :

1. *Causes in relation to soul* : *Papa,* i.e. sins of past life of the individual and of parents are responsible for foetal abnormalities and idiopathic diseases.

2. *Hereditary factors* : Gross defects in sperms or ova give, rise to sterility or abortion. Defective chromosomes and

genes, i.e. *bija-bhagavayava* are responsible for abnormalities of sex organs.

3. *Consanguinity* : It is important to avoid marriage in close relatives as the chances of inheriting. Hereditary diseases are increased. Hereditary diseases like diabetes are incurable.

4. *Age of parents* : The seeds in man and woman mature at the age of twenty five and sixteen respectively. If parents are below this age, the foetus does not develop, dies early or becomes deformed.

5. Intercourse in an abnormal posture leads to a deformed child.

6. *Increased doshas* : Increased *Vata, Pitta* and *Kapha* in the foetus lead to congenital anomalies. Increase *Vata,* i.e. *Vataprakopaka* gives rise to a deformed, deaf and dumb child and paralysis.

7. *Constitution* : Both the parents should not have the same disease, constitutions, e.g. if both the parents have *Kapha* constitution, the offspring is likely to have *Kaphaja* diseases like congenital turnouts.

8. *Constitution based on basic elements* : The constitution of both the parents should not be dominant in the same basic clement, e. g. if the energy element is dominant in both the parents, the fetus is likely to suffer from *Pitta* constitution and anomalies of the eyes including blindness. On tlle other hand, if the energy element is weak in both the parents, marked decrease or absence of energy element will again give rise to blindness. If the energy element accompanies blood, *Pitta* or *Kapha* of the foetus in excess, the colour of the iris will be red, brown or white respectively. If the energy element joins *Vata*, it leads to a squint in the foetus.

9. Not fulfilling the demands and cravings of the pregnant lady arising from the tissue demands of mother and child. Effect of some of the maternal cravings on the foetus are given in the following Table :

Craving in mother	Effect on foetus
• Seeing the king	Lucky and rich person
• Wearing slik or woolen clothes or ornaments.	Child or person develop a liking for ornaments and enjoyments
• Seeing idols of God	Person with good character
• Visiting hermitage of saints	Religious and having control over his sense organs
• Seeing cruel animals like tigers	Indulging in violence
• Eating :	
(a) Flesh of godha	Sleepy and good runer
(b) Cow's flesh	Strong and able to bear stress and strains of various types
(c) Buffalo's flesh	Brave, hairy and having red eyes
(d) Pig's flesh	Brave and sleepy
(e) Deer's flesh	Carries out call the activities with speed and enjoys living in jungles
(f) Cow residing in jungle	Depressed
(g) Flesh of *tittira* bird	Fearful

10. If mother's diet is excessively hot, heavy and pungent, it is injurious to the infant. The details are given in the following table. Eating too less a diet may lead to foetal malnutrition.

11. *Activities* : Abnormal activities and riding on animals for a long time, as given in the following table may be harmful to the foetus :

Mother's diet and activity in pregnancy	Effects on the foetus or on characters of the child
• Sleeping in prone position	Loops of cord round the neck
• Travelling in excess all the time	Loops of cord round the neck
• Sleeping alone in open place or wandering alone at night	Insance Child
• Indulges in falsehood and quarelling with other	Epilepsy

Mother's diet and activity in pregnancy	Effects on the foetus or on characters of the child
• Excessive indulgence in sex	Congenital abnoramalites, epilepsy, sexy and shameless
• Remains in a sorrowfel state	Fearfrl and thin child and with a short life-span
• Jealous of others	Jealous, cruel or dominated by his wife
• Commits theft	Hard working, jealous and undertaking bad deeds
• Angry	Angry, unreliable and criticisng others
• Sleeping in excess	Sleepy, foolish and with weak digestive power
• Drinking alcohol in excess regularly	Thirsty with wavering mind and weak memory
• Likes and eats flesh of *godha*	Stones in urinary tract and difficult in passing urine, sleepy
• Likes pig's flesh	Red eyes, crying in excess and having rough hair brave, sleepy
• Eating fish in excess regularly	Infrequent blinking and fixed eyes
• Eating sweet food items in excess	Large sized, dumb and diadetic child
• Eating in excess salty food items	Early wrinking of skin, bladness and early greying of hair
• Eating in excess sour food items	Bleeding disorders, skin or eye diseases
• Eating in excess pungent food items	Weak, sterile and weak sexual powers
• Eating in excess bitter food items	Emaciation or tuberculosis weak or ugly looking
• Eating in excess astringent food items	Dark complexion, distension of abdomen and intestinal obstruction
• Medicinal smoking for fever	Blindness, weakness or abortion
Indulgence in diet and activity promoting	
(a) *Vata*	Blind, deformed, short and dull
(b) *Pitta*	Brown colour and faulters
(c) *Kapha*	Pallor and leucoderma

(12) Local injury to abdomen may damage the foetus.

(13) Diseases and infections in mother may damage the foetus.

(14) Suppression of natural urges, particularly of passing urine, stool and wind may be harmful to the foetus. It will increase *Vata* in the mother, which in turn increase *Vata* in the foetus giving rise to *Vataja* anomalies.

(15) Use of sense organs in an abnormal manner :

   (a) Hearing unpleasant words or distressing news, hearing shrill noises may lead to deafness in the foetus.

   (b) Looking at water fall for a long time may be harmful to the foctus.

(16) Iatrogenic causes (*pancakarma*), i. e. induction of sweating, emesis, purgation, enema, cleansing nasal medications and administering hot drugs to the mother may lead to abortion, discolouration or a congenital anomaly.

(17) Non-religious conduct of the parents and mother's act of not observing regulations prior to the menstrual period may be harmful to the foetus as given in the following table. The practices advised by religion during menstrual period are important, as deviation from these prescribed practices will have maximum influence on the maturing ovum, which is released from the ovarian surface. In addition, it will have little influence over other germinal cells and ova.

   Results of violation of the rules and regulations to be followed by the lady during menstrual period :

Violation of rules by the lady during menstrual period	Effect on the fetus and Child
• Clipping nails during periods	Abnormalities of nails
• Oil Massage	Chronic skin diseases
• Personal make-up	
(a) Application of scents and powder	Leads a miserable life
(b) Eye ointmental-*kajal* and wearing ornaments	Blindness

Violation of rules by the lady during menstrual period	Effect on the fetus and Child
● Bath	Leads a miserable life
● Sleep during day	Excessive sleep
● Running	Unsteady, unstable
● Talking in excess	Talkative
● Laughing loudly in excess	Blackish discoloration of lips, teeth and palate
● Digging earth	Faulters
● Exertion	Uncontrolled activity and behaviour
● Hearing loud sounds	Deafness
● Exposure to breeze	Uncontrolled behaviour and activity
● Weeping and crying	Abnormalities of eyes

(18) *Psychological factors* : Increased *raja* and *tama* qualities of mind give rise to personality disorders. Getting angry and jealous can also lead to congenital anomalies.

(19) *Addiction* : Drinking alcohol in excess and smoking heavily, during pregnancy can have adverse effects on the foetus. It can lead to congenital anomalies in the foetus.

MANIFESTATIONS

Damage to the foetus and to the mother is indicated if the pregnant lady develops following signs and symptoms :

(1) Develops fever, weakness and pallor.

(2) Eats in excess and continues to eat till she faints.

(3) Develops prominent eyes, cold limbs and ears and knotted hair.

(4) Has a foetus that lies entirely above the umbilicus.

(5) Develops arthritis and septic foci in the body and finds difficulty in walking.

(6) Is worried too much or suffers from sorrow.

(7) Has foul-smelling milk and develops knotting of hair.

(8) Develops cyanosis and generalised oedema.

(9) Develops backache, thirst, breathlessness and unconsciousness.

(10) Develops pain in the waist and vagina, foul-smelling breath, delirium and unconsciousness.

(11) Develops nystagmus, stiff nose and smells like that of bird.

(12) Smells like that of a goat or horse, craves for peacock's flesh and becomes pale.

(13) Wears red dress, red garlands, laughs in sleep and walks towards a cemetry.

(14) Dreams of riding on ass, pig, buffalo, dog or camel.

In these cases it is better to induce abortion or miscarriage or remove the foetus by surgical means and save the life of the mother.

Apart from the various congenital anomalies mentioned earlier, congenital anomalies of sexual organs are also described in Ayurvedic texts. They are :

(1) *Dvireta* : when the foetus, i.e. child manifests both the male and female, genital organs, i.e. true hermaphrodite.

(2) *Rantha or Varta* : Defect in the genes of the genital organs in the female. Depending on the severity, she may be sterile, have abortion or have none of the qualities of the female.

(3) *Truna putrika or Truna pulika or Trunamukha* : Defect in the genes of the genital organs in the male. Depending on the severity of the defect, he may be sterile or many not have any quality of the male.

(4) *Nara Shandha* : Such a male preson looks like and behaves like a female. Such a person is born, if during intercourse father lies in supine and mother takes active part in the intercourse. The sperms are absent.

(5) *Narishandha* : Such a female behaves like a male and enjoys sexual union with another female, ovaries are absent.

(6) *Anasthi Vatika Shandha* : Undescended testes or absence of testes, both of which lead to sterility.

(7) *Pavanendriya* : Here *Vata* destroys the seminal vesicles in the male. Hence, he is a sterile person though potent.

PREVENTION

It is important to avoid aetiological factors of hereditary and congenital diseases. The natural desires and cravings of the pregnant women arise from the tissue demand of the foetus and mother. The desire to eat earth is seen in pregnant women, who has iron deficiency anaemia and this desire represents nature's attempt to get the iron from earth. It is better to give a particular item which the pregnant women longs for, unless it is dangerous to the foetus. In such a case innocuous item resembling the item craved for should be given in a disguised form. If cravings of the pregnant women are not fulfilled, it often leads to *Vataprakopa* and the foetus may become deformed, deaf, dumb and may develop paralysis.

To prevent congenital anomalies, the pregnant women should avoid : (i) Unhappy state of mind or getting upset if the desires are not fulfiled, (ii) Anything that might injure her sense or motor orgnas, (iii) Anything that experienced women and physicians declare as harmful, (iv) Wearing red clothes, (v) Taking intoxicating wines, (vi) Travelling in a carriage, (vii) Violent-movements, (viii) Heavy, hot and pungent food items, (ix) Anything to which the pregnant women is not habituated, and (x) Inadequate or unbalanced diet, which would affect the nutrition.

It is important to avoid aetiological factors of hereditary diseases and congenital anomalies. Atharvaveda mentions the use of *bhagavati*, i.e. *laghushatavari, aparajita* or *vishnukranta* and *taraka*, i.e. *indravaruni* by expectant parents and pregnant ladies for the prevention of hereditary diseases. For the prevention of congenital heart disease, the pregnant lady should take *mrigshrin-gabhasma.*

The monthly regime of diet and medicine; to be followed by a pregnant lady as given in the chapter 19 of Balaveda are also worth trying. It is worth-while trying certain religious rites like *putreshti yajna* as prescribed by the scriptures.

जन्मबलप्रवृत्त व्याधय:

बीजभागदोष:

शुक्रस्य दोषात् क्लैब्यमहर्षणम् ।

रोगी वा क्लीबमल्पायुर्विरूपं वा प्रजायते ।।

न चास्य जायते गर्भ: पतति प्रस्त्रवत्यपि ।

शुक्रं हि दुष्टं सापत्यं सदारं बाधते नरम् ।।   (च.सू. 28/18-19)

यदि च मनुष्यो मनुष्यप्रभव:, कस्मान् जडादिभ्यो जाता: पितृसदृशरूपा भवन्तीति; तत्रोच्यते यस्य यस्य ह्यङ्गावयवस्य बीजे बीजभाग उपतप्तो भवति, तस्य तस्याङ्गावयवस्य विकृतिरूपजायते, नोपजायते चानुपतापात्; तस्मादुभयोपपत्तिरप्यत्र । सर्वस्य चात्मजानी इन्द्रियाणि, तेषां भावाभावहेतुर्दैवं तस्मान्नैकान्ततो जडादिभ्यो जाता: पितृसदृशरूपा: भवन्ति ।।   (च.शा. 3/17)

गर्भोपघातकरा: भावा:

गर्भोपघातकरास्त्विमे भावा: भवन्ति:; तद्यथा-सर्वमतिगुरुष्णतीक्ष्ण दारुणाश्च चेष्ठा:, इमांश्चान्यानुपदिशन्ति वृद्धा:-देवतारक्षोऽनुचरपरिरक्षणार्थ न रक्तानि वासांसि बिभृयात्र मदकराणि मद्यान्यभ्यवहदून यानमधिरोहेन्न मांसमश्नीयात् सर्वेन्द्रिय प्रतिकूलांश्च भावान् दूरत: परिवर्जयेत् । यच्चान्यदपि किञ्चित् स्त्रीयो विदु: ।

(च.शा. 4/18)

मात्रादीनामेव तु खलु गर्भकराणां भावानां व्यापत्तिनिमित्तस्याजन्म भवति ।

ये ह्यस्य कुक्षौ वृद्धिहेतुसमाख्याता भावास्तेषां विपर्ययादुदरे विनाशमापद्यते, अथवाप्यचिरजात: स्यात् ।   (च.शा. 4/28-29)

एवमेव पुरुषस्य यदा बीजे बीजभाग: प्रदोषमापद्यते, तदा वन्ध्यं जनयति; यदा पुनरस्य बीजे बीजभागावयव: प्रदोषमापद्यते तदा पूतिप्रजं जनयति, यदा त्वस्य बीजे बीजभागावयव: पुरुषकराणां च शरीरबीजभागानामेकदेश: प्रदोषमापद्यते, तदा

पुरुषाकृतिभूयिष्ठमपुरुषं तृणपत्रिकं नाम जनयति तां पुरुषव्यापादमा चक्षते।

(च. शा. 4/131)

एतेन मातृजानां पितृजानां चावयवानां विकृतिव्याख्यानेन सात्म्यजानां रसजानां सत्त्वजाना चावयवानां विकृतिर्व्याख्याता भवति। (च. शा. 4/32)

निर्विकार: परस्त्वात्मा सर्वभूतानां निर्विशेष:; सत्त्वशरीरयोस्तु विशेषाद् विशेषोपलब्धि:। (च. शा. 4/33)

तत्र त्रय: शरीरदोषा वातपित्तश्लेष्माण:, ते शरीरं दूषयन्ति; द्वौ पुन: सत्त्वदोषौ रजस्तमश्च तौ सत्त्वं दूषयत:। ताभ्यां च सत्त्वशरीराभ्यां दुष्टाभ्यां विकृतिरूपजायते, नोपजायते चाप्रदुष्टाभ्याम्। (च. शा. 4/34)

तत ऋत्विक् प्रागुत्तरस्यां दिश्यगारस्य प्राक्प्रवणमुदक्प्रवणं वा प्रदेशमभिसमीक्ष्य, गोमयोदकाभ्यां स्थण्डिलमुपलिप्य, प्रोक्ष्य चोदकेन, वेदीमस्मिन् स्थापयेत्। तां पश्चिमेनानाहतवस्त्रसञ्चये श्वेतार्षभे वाऽप्यजिन उपविशेद् ब्राह्मणप्रयुक्त:, राजन्यप्रयुक्तस्तु वैयाघ्रेचर्मण्यानदुहे वा, वैश्यप्रयुक्तस्तु रौरवे वास्ते वा। तत्रोपविष्ट: पालाशीभिरैन्दुदीभिरौदुम्बरीभिर्माधूकीभिर्वा समिद्भिरग्निमुपसमाधाय, कुशै: परिस्तीर्य परिधिभिश्च परिधाय लाजै: शुक्लाभिश्च गन्धवतीभि: सुमनोभिरुपकिरेत्। तत्र प्रणीयोदपात्रं पवित्रपूतमुपसंस्कृत्य सर्पिराज्यार्थं यथोक्तवर्णानाजानेयादीन् समन्तत: स्थापयेत्। (च. शा. 8/10)

अत ऊर्ध्वं गर्भस्थापनानि व्याख्यास्याम:-ऐन्द्री ब्राह्मी शतवीर्या सहस्रवीर्याऽमोघा-ऽव्यथा शिवाष्यऽरिष्टा वाट्यपुष्पी विष्वक्सेनकन्ता चेत्यासामोषधीनां शिरसा दक्षिणेन वा पाणिना धारणम्, एताभिश्चैव सिद्धस्य पयस: सर्पिषो वा पानम्, एताभिश्चैव पुष्पे पुष्पे स्नानं सदा च ता: समालभेत। तथा सर्वासां जीवनीयोक्तानामोषधीनां सदोपयोगस्तैरूपयोगविधिभि:। इति गर्भस्थापनानि व्याख्यातानि भवन्ति। (च. शा. 8/20)

गर्भोपघातकरास्त्विमे भावा भवन्ति; तद्यथा-उत्कटविषमकठिनासनसेविन्या वातमूत्रपरीषवेगानुपरुन्धत्या दारुणानुचितव्यायामसेविन्यास्तीक्ष्णोष्णातिमात्रसेविन्या: प्रमिताशनसेविन्या गर्भ म्रियतेऽन्त: कुक्षे:, अकाले वा स्रंसते, शोषीऽवा भवति; तथाऽभिघातप्रपीडने: श्वभ्रकूपप्रपातदेशावलोकनैर्वाऽभीक्ष्णं मातु: प्रपत्यकाले गर्भ:; तथाऽतिमात्रसङ्क्षोभिभिर्यानैर्नयनैर्न, अप्रियातिमात्रश्रवणैर्वा। प्रततोत्तानशयिन्या: पुनर्गर्भस्य नाभ्याश्रया नाडी कण्ठमनुवेष्ट्यति, विवृतशायिनी नक्तंचारिणी चोन्मत्तं जनयति, अपस्मारिणं पुन: कलिकलहशीला, व्यावायशीला दुर्वपुषमह्रीकं स्त्रैणं वा शोकनित्या भीतमपचितमल्पायुषं वा, अभिध्यात्री परोच्चतापिनमीर्ष्युं स्त्रैणं वा, स्तेना

त्वायासबहुलमतिद्रोहिणमकर्मशीलं वा, अमर्षिणी चण्डमौपधिकमसूयकं वा, स्वप्ननित्या तन्द्रालुमबुधमल्पर्ज्जिनं वा, मद्यनित्या पिपासालुमल्पस्मृतिमनवस्थितचित्तं वा, गोधामांसप्राया शार्करिणमश्मरिणं शनैर्मेहिणं वा। वराहमांसप्राया रक्ताक्षं क्रथनमतिपरुषरोमाणं वा, मत्स्यामांसनित्या चिरनिमेषं स्तब्धाक्षं, वा मधुरनित्या प्रमेहिणं मूकमतिस्थूलं वा, अम्लनित्या रक्तपित्तिनं त्वगक्षिरोगिणं वा, लवणनित्या शीघ्रव-लीपलितं खालित्यरोगिणं वा, कटुकनित्या दुर्बलमल्पशुक्रमनपत्यं वा, तिक्तनित्या शोषिणमबलमनुचितं वा, कषायनित्या श्यावमानाहिनमुदावर्तिनं वा, यद्यच्च यस्य यस्य व्याधेर्निदानमुक्तं तत्तदासेवमानाऽन्तर्वत्नी तन्निमित्तविकारबहुलमपत्यं जनयति। पितृजास्तु शुक्रदोषा मातृजैरपचारैर्व्याख्याता:। इति गर्भोपघातकरा: भावा भवन्त्युक्ता:।

(च. शा. 8)

तस्मादहितानाहारविहारान् प्रजासम्पदमिच्छन्ती स्त्री विशेषण वर्जयेत्। साध्वाचारा चात्मानमुपचरेद्धिताभ्याहारविहाराभ्यामिति।   (च. शा. 8/21)

व्याधींश्चास्या मृदुमधुरशिशिरसुखसुकुमारप्रायैषधाहारोपचारैरूपचरेत्, न चास्या वमनविरेचनशिरोविरेचनानि प्रयोजयेत्, न रक्तमवसेचयेत्, सर्वकालं च नास्थापन-मनुवासनं वा कुर्यादन्यत्रात्ययिकाद् व्याधे:। अष्टमं मासमुपादाय वमनादिसाध्येषु पुनर्विकारेष्वात्ययिकेषु मृदुभिर्वमनादिभिस्तदर्थकारिभिर्वोपचार: स्यात्। पूर्णमिव तैलपात्रमसंक्षोभयताऽन्तर्वत्नी भवत्युपचर्या।   (च. शा. 8/22)

सा चेदपचारद् द्वयोस्त्रिषु वा मासेषु पुष्पं पश्येन्नास्या गर्भ:। स्थास्यतीति विद्यात्; अजातसारो हि तस्मिन् काले भवति गर्भ:।   (च. शा. 8/23)

सा चेच्चयतुष्प्रभृतिषु मासेषु क्रोधशोकासूयेष्यर्ष्याभयत्रासव्यवायव्यायामसंक्षोभसन्धारण-विषमाशनशयनस्थानक्षुत्पिपासानियोगात् कदाहारद् वा पुष्पं पश्येत्, तस्या गर्भस्थापन-विधिमुपदेक्ष्याम्। पुष्पदर्शनादेवैनां ब्रूयात्–शयनं तावन्मृदुसुखशिशिरास्तरणसंस्ती-र्णमीषदवनतशिरस्कं प्रतिपद्यस्वेति। ततो यष्टीमधुकसर्पिभ्यां परमशिशिरवारिणी संस्थिताभ्यां पिचुमाप्लाव्योपस्थसमीपे स्थापयेत् तस्या:, तथा शतधौत सहस्रधौताभ्यां सर्पिम्याम्यधोनाभे: सर्वत: प्रदिह्यात्, सर्वतश्च गव्येन चैनां पयसा सुशीतेन मधुकाम्बुना वा न्यग्रोधादिकषयेण वा परिषेचयेदधो नाभे:; उदकं सुशीतमवगाहयेत्, क्षीरिणां कषादुमाणां च स्वरसपरिपीतानि चेलानि ग्राहयेत्, न्यग्रोधादि शुङ्ग सिद्धयोर्वा क्षीरसर्पिषो: पिचुं ग्राहयेत्, अतश्चैवाक्षमात्रं प्राशयेत्, प्राशयेद् वा केवलं क्षीरसर्पि:, पद्मोत्पलकुमुदकिञ्जल्कांश्चास्यै समधुशर्करान् लेहार्थं दद्यात्, शृङ्गाटकपुष्करबीज कशेरुकान् भक्षणार्थं, गन्धप्रियङ्गुसितोत्पलशालूकोदुम्बरशलाटुन्यग्रोधशुङ्गानि वा पाययेदेनामाजेन पयसा, पयसा चैनां बलातिबलाशलिषष्टिकेक्षुमूलकाकोली श्रृतेन समधुशर्करं रक्तशालीनामोदनं मृदुसुरभिशीतलं भोजयेत्, लावकपिञ्जल-

कुरङ्गशम्बरशशहरिणैणकालपुच्छकरसेन वा घृतेसुसंकृतेन सुखशिशिरोपवातदेशस्थां
भोजयेत् क्रोधशोकायाससव्यवायव्यायामेभ्यश्चाभिरक्षेत्, सौम्याभिश्चैनां
कथाभिर्मनोनुकूलाभिरूपासित; तथाऽस्या गर्भस्तिष्ठति । (च. शा. 8/24)

यस्या: पुनरामान्वयात् पुष्पदर्शनं स्यात् प्रायस्तस्यास्तद् गर्भोपघातकरं भवति,
विरुद्धोपक्रमत्वात् तयो: । (च. शा. 8/25)

जात: प्रमेही मधुमेहिनी वा न साध्य उक्त: स हि बीजदोषात् ।

ये चापि केचित् कुलजा विकारा भवन्ति तांश्च प्रवदन्त्यसाध्यान् । (च.चि. 6/57)

कुर्णिर्वा यदि वाऽन्धश्च जायते दुर्बलेन्द्रिय: ।

धूम्रपानेन गार्भिण्या धूमतेजोहतो भृशम् ।।

विवर्णो जायते गर्भ: पतेद्वाऽपि विशांपते । (काश्यप-खिलस्थान-10/20)

ततु सप्तविधे व्याधावुपनिपतति । ते पुन: सप्तविधा व्याधय: । तद्यथा-आदिबलप्रवृत्ता:,
जन्मबलप्रवृत्ता:, दोषबलप्रवृत्ता:, सङ्घातबलप्रवृत्ता:, कालबलप्रवृत्ता:, दैवबलप्रवृत्ता:,
स्वभावबलप्रवृत्ता: इति । (सु. सू. 24/5)

बीजेऽन्तर्वायुना भिन्ने द्वौ जीवौ कुक्षिमागतौ ।

यमावित्यभिदीयेते धर्मेतरपुरस्सरौ ।।

पित्रोरत्यल्पबीजत्वदासेक्य: पुरुषो भवेत् ।

स शुक्रं प्राश्य लभते ध्वजोच्छ्रयमसंशयम् ।।

य: पूतियोनौ जायेत स सौगन्धिकसञ्ज्ञित: ।

स योनिशेफसोर्गन्धमाघ्राय लभते बलम् ।।

स्वे गुदेऽब्रह्मचर्याद्च: स्त्रीषु पुंवत् प्रवर्तते ।

कुम्भीक: स तु विज्ञेय: ·················· ।।

··············ईर्ष्यकं शृणु चापरम् ।

दृष्ट्वा व्यवायमन्येषां व्यवाये य: प्रवर्तते ।।

ईर्ष्यक: स च विज्ञेय:·············· ।।

··············षण्डकं शृणु पञ्चमम् ।

यो भार्यायामृतौ मोहादङ्गनेव प्रवर्तते ।

तत: स्त्रीचेष्टिताकारो जायते षण्डसञ्ज्ञित: ।।

ऋतौ पुरुषवद्वाऽपि प्रवर्त्तेताङ्गना यदि ।

तत्र कन्या यदि भवेत् सा भवेन्नरचेष्टिता।।

आसेक्यश्च सुगन्धी च कुम्भीकश्चेर्ष्यकस्तथा।
सरेतसस्त्वमी ज्ञेया अशुक्र: षण्डसञ्ज्ञित:।।

अनया विप्रकृत्या तु तेषां शुक्रवहा: सिरा:।
हर्षात् स्फुटत्वमायान्ति ध्वजोच्छ्रयस्ततो भवेत्।।

आहाराचारचेष्टाभिर्यादृशीभि: समन्वितौ।
स्त्रीपुंसौ समुपेयातां तयो: पुत्रोऽपि तादृश:।।

यदा नार्यावुपेयातां वृषस्यन्त्यौ कथञ्चन।
मुञ्चान्त्यौ शुक्रमन्योऽन्यमनस्थितस्तत्र जायते।।

ऋतुस्नाता तु या नारी स्वप्ने मैथुनमावहेत्।
आर्त्तवं वायुरादाय कुक्षौ गर्भं करोति हि।।

मासि मासि विवर्द्धेत गर्भिण्या गर्भलक्षणम्।
कललं जायते तस्या वर्जितं पैतृकैर्गुणै:।।

सर्पवृश्चिककूष्माण्डविकृताकृतयश्च ये।
गर्भास्त्वेते सित्रयाश्चैव ज्ञेया: पापकृतो भृशम्।।

गर्भो वातप्रकोपेण द्रौहृदे वाऽवमानिते।
भवेत् कुब्ज: कुणि: पङ्गुर्मूको मिन्मिनेव वा।।

मातापित्रोस्तु नास्तिक्यादशुभैश्च पुराकृतै:।
वातादीनां प्रकोपेण गर्भो वैकृतमाप्नुयात्।।   (सु. शा. 2/40-55)

सन्निपातजानि सर्वदोषलक्षणयुक्तानि।।   (सु. नि. 2/15)

स्त्रीपुंसयो: कुष्ठदोषाद् दुष्टशोणितशुक्रयो:।
यदपत्यं तजोर्जातं ज्ञेयं तदापि कुष्ठितम्।।   (सु. नि. 5/27)

कृमिवातभिघातैस्तु तदेवोपद्रुतं फलम्।
पतत्यकालेऽपि यथा तथा स्याद् गर्भविच्युति:।।

आचतुर्थात्ततो मासात् प्रस्रवेद् गर्भविच्युति:।
तत: स्थिरशरीरस्य पात: पञ्चमषष्ठयो:।।

प्रविध्यति शिरो या तु शीताङ्गी निरपत्रपा।

नीलोद्धत सिरा हन्ति सा गर्भं स च तां तथा।।

गर्भास्पन्दनमावीनां प्रणाश: श्यावपाण्डुता।

भवत्युच्छ्वासपुतित्वं शूलं चान्तमृते शिशौ।।

भानसागन्तुभिर्मातुरूपतापै: प्रपीडित:।

गर्भो व्यापद्यते कुक्षौ व्याधिभिश्च प्रपीडित:।।

बस्तमारविपन्नाया: कुक्षि: प्रस्पन्दते यदि।

तत्क्षणात्जन्मकाले तं पाटयित्वोद्धरेद्भिषक्।।   (सु. नि. 8/11–16)

निरुद्धप्रकशे तस्मिन् मन्दधारमवेदनम्।

मूत्रं प्रवर्तते जन्तोर्मणिर्न च विदीर्यते।।

निरुद्धप्रकशं विद्यात् सरुजं वातसम्भवम्।।   (सु. नि. 13/55–56)

निषिद्धोपक्रमसेविन्या: सगभर्भाया: विकारचिकित्सा

स्त्रीचेदापन्नगर्भा परिहार्याण्यासेवेत। तत्र यस्या बस्तिपार्श्वश्रोणियोनिमुखेषु शूलं पुष्पदर्शनं वा स्यात्।

तां मृदुसुखशिशिरास्तरणशयनस्थामीषदवनतिशिरसं शीतप्रमेहपरिषेकादिभिरूपाचरेत्।

(अं. सं. शा. 4/3)

गर्भिणी वर्ज्य कर्माणि

अतिव्यवायमायासं भारं प्रावरणं गुरु।

अकालजागरस्वप्नं कठिनोत्कटकासनम्।।

शीकक्रोधभयोद्वेगवेगश्रद्धाविधारणम्।

उपवासाध्वतीक्ष्णोष्णगुरुविष्टम्भिभोजनम्।।

रक्तं निवसनं शवभ्रकूपेक्षां मद्यमामिषम्।

उत्तानशयनं यच्च स्त्रियो नेच्छन्ति तत्त्यजेत्।।

तथा रक्तस्रुतिं शुद्धि वस्तिमामासतोऽष्टमात्।

एभिर्गर्भः स्रवेदाम: कुक्षौ शुष्येन्म्रियेत वा।।   (अ. हृ. शा. 1/44–47)

4

SUPPRESSION OF NATURAL URGES
(VEGAVARODHA)

For biological existence and optimum functioning, every individual requires a continuous supply of food, water and air. He must excrete the waste products which are being continuously formed as a result of metabolic activities. He must take rest intermittently to replenish the loss incurred during activity. Desires or urges to fulfil these biological needs are naturally present in every individual in the form of hunger, thirst, micturition, defaecation, sleep, etc.

Suppression as well as induction of biological urges are important causes of several diseases or their symptoms. The biological urges arc classified as :

(1) Urge for elimination or excretion of waste products :
    (i) Solid waste products (Stools)
    (ii) Liquid waste products
       (a) Micturition (Urine) (b) Emesis (Vomitus).
    (iii) Gaseous waste products :
       (a) Passage of wind through anus, (b) belching,
       (c) Exertional breathlessness, (d) Yawning.
(2) Protective reflexes which are meant to keep the air passages clear :
    (i) Sneezing, (ii) Coughing.
(3) Natural secretions :
    (i) Semen (Ejaculation)
    (ii) Tears (Following sorrow or happiness)

(4) Urges for self survival :

   (i) Hunger (Eating food)

   (ii) Thirst (Drinking water)

   (iii) Sleep (Rest)

Charaka and Vagbhata have described these entities under the chapter on suppression of biological urges. But Sushruta includes them under the chapter on *udavarta*. The word *udavarta* signifies that following suppression of biological urges, the natural flow of impulses tends to spread in the reverse, upward or abnormal direction. Apart from suppression of biological urges, mechanical or nervous causes like anal stenosis can give rise to the same symptom complex. All mechanical conditions, neurologic causes and other conditions included under the term *udavarta* are not discussed in this chapter.

All the urges are controlled by nervous system, i.e. *Vata*. Suppression or induction of biological urges both result in increased irritability of nervous system and *Vataprakopa*. Suppression of urges in addition results in retention of waste products and toxemia giving rise to severe and chronic diseases, which may be dangerous to life, if not controlled in time. The retained waste products also predispose a person to secondary infection. As an example the pathogenesis of the symptoms complex following suppression of micturition is given below. Suppression of micturition results in retention of urine and distension of bladder. If there is obstruction to the outflow this can as well lead to evolution of some symptoms complex.

Artificial induction of micturition may increase the irritability of bladder and lead to local symptoms like dysuria. However, it will not give rise to general symptoms or predispose a person to sepsis. Suppression of biological urge, i.e. *vegavarodha* is much more harmful than artificial induction of the urge *vegodirana*. Hence, emphasis is laid on suppression rather than induction of biological urges as a cause of disease.

Suppression of Passage of Gas through Anus : Suppression of wind, i.e. *apana vayu* gives rise to colicky pain, constipation and distension. It may occasionally give rise to paralytic ileus and result in mucous, bilious and later faecal vomiting. If chronic, it may result in *gulma* (cystic abdominal lump).

Suppression of this reflex and distended rectum results in retention of urine and distension of bladder. Beecause of distension it gives rise to hiccup, breathlessness and pain in the cardiac region. If habitual or chronic, by affecting general health, it predisposes a person to develop recurrent cold, cough, pharyngitis, *asthma* and heart disease. The toxic products after absorption give rise to headache, heaviness of the body, bodyache, exhaustion and diminished clarity of vision.

Treatment : The patient should be given medicated oil or ghee by mouth and sweating should be induced later. Suppositories and enemas are helpftil. The patient should take diet which will enhance normal peristaltic activity of intestines and colon and drink lukewarm water.

Suppression of Defaecation : Suppression of defaecation gives rise to cutting pain in the ano-rectal, region, colicky pain in colon and abdomen, retention of faeces and gases, distension of abdomen, gurgling noises in abdomen, belching and difficulty in passing wind or stools. Occasionally it may result in faecal vomiting or *gulma* which is a cystic type of abdominal lump.

Because of pressure of retained faeces and gases on adjacent it organs, gives rise to retention of urine, breathlessness and pain in the cardiac region. If chronic, it may lead to chronic cold, *asthma* and heart disease. The waste products after absorption give rise to headache, muscle cramps, bodyache and exhaustion.

Treatment : Suppositories and enema are useful. The patient should sit in a tub containing a decoction of drugs, which would subdue *Vata*. The patient should be massaged with oil. This should be followed by induction of sweating. If distension is present, the patient should fast and then vomiting is induced if necessary. Later, the patient should be given light diet like yava *(java)*, buttermilk, vegetables like *vastuka* which would also help to split the dry, scybalous, retained faeces. In addition, one should administer digestives and drugs, which would subdue *Vata* and increase secretion of digestive juice In general, one should follow the treatment of distension of abdomen, i.e. *anaha*.

Suppression of Micturition : Suppressed micturition gives rise to retention of urine, pain in bladder, penis and tesis, distension of lower abdomen and dysuria. The patient may be unable to pass urine due to over-distension of bladder and later develop urinary incontinence. Suppression of the reflex and distended bladder by its pressure-effect gives rise to retention of faeces and gases, distension, pain around umbilicus and if chronic may lead to *gulma*, i.e. cystic abdominal lump like hydrone-phrosis. Distension may also lead to breathlessness (acidosis), cough, exhaustion and diminished clarity of vision.

Tub bath, oil massage, induction of sweating, enemas and bladder was are important therapeutic measures. The patient should be given *avapidanasneha,* i.e. medicated ghee in good quantity before meals and after food is digested. One should avoid oil administration orally as *tila* oil gives rise to constipation and oliguria.

The following remedies should be tried for suppressed micturition :

   (i) Wine should be mixed with milk, cardamom or large quantity of *souvarchala* salt and taken.

  (ii) The juice of *dhatri* or *amalaka* (Indian goose berry) diluted with water should be taken daily for three days.

 (iii) Cooked meat should be taken with honey and wine prepared from jaggery or grapes.

 (iv) One *tola*, i.e. three teaspoonfuls of compound powder consisting of *bhadradaru, musta, murva, haridra* and

yashtimadhu should be dissolved in adequate quantity
of rain water and then taken.

(v)   The expressed juice of *duralabha*, i.e. *dusparsha* or
decoction of *arujna* or saffron should taken.

(vi) Seeds of cucumber mixed with a little salt should be
taken with water.

(vii) *Panchamula* or dry black grapes cooked in milk is
useful.

(viii) Medicines prescribed for dysuria or bladder stone or
obstruction of urine like *shilaiatu, shatavari ghrita,
gokshuradi quath* are useful.

Suppression of Vomiting : Suppression of vomiting gives
rise to nausea, anorexia, fever, anaemia oedema, cough, breathlessness, eye diseases and skin diseases like *kushtha, vyanga,
visarpa* and *kotha.*

Treatment : Oil medicated with salt should be used for
massaging and medicated ghee should given internally. Vomiting
should be induced after administration of some food. After emesis
the patient should fast for few hours and later take light the dry
diet. Gargling, smoking cigarettes prepared from herbs having
antiemetic action, exercise, purgatives and blood letting are useful
therapeutic measures.

Supression of Cough : Suppression of cough results in
increased bouts of cough, breathlessness, and hiccup. It also leads
to anorexia, emaciation and heart disease (Cor pulmonale).

Treatment consists of administration of medicines and
measures described for *kasa,* i.e. cough.

Suppression of Sneezing : Suppression of sneezing leads
to diseases of nose, pharynx, larynx, ears, eyes and head. It gives
rise to sense of fullness and pain in the mouth and throat, noisy
respiration, headache, hemicrania, weakness of sense organs,
stiffness of neck and facial paralysis (following otitis media).

Treatment consists of oil massage, administration of

medicated oil or ghee, induction of sweating and sneezing. Sneezing is induced by strong nose drops, smoking strong medicated cigarettes, stimulating mucosa of nose by a cotton wick, looking at the Sun, strong eye ointments or snuff with strong smell. The patient should take ghee after meals.

Suppression of Exertional Breathlessness : Suppression of exertional breathlessness leads to fainting, heart disease and emphysema. The treatment consists of rest, administration of mutton soup and measures to subdue the increased *Vata*.

Suppression of Yawning : Suppression of yawning like sneezing gives rise to diseases of mouth, throat, nose, ear, eyes and head. It gives rise to stretching or contraction of body, stiffness of neck and thighs, tremors, convulsions, headache, drowsiness and facial paralysis. The treatment consists of giving medicated oil or ghee, induction of sweating and other therapeutic measures to subdue the increased *Vata*.

Suppression of Belching : When belching is suppressed, one develops anorexia, fullness of mouth and throat, distension of stomach, constipation, hiccup, cough, breathlessness, and sense of constriction in the chest. The increased *Vata (Vata prakopa)* gives rise to tremors, severe body pains and severe illness due to disorders of *Vata*. The treatment consists of smoking unctuous medicated cigarettes and administration of wine with lemon juice and *souvarchala* salt–both of which induce belching. In general, one should follow the treatment of hiccup.

Suppression of Ejaculation : Suppression of sex urge results in pain and swelling of penis, scrotum and bladder. It may result in retention of urine, inguinal hernia, prostatic calculi and involuntary discharge of semen. Chronic suppression may result in splitting body-ache, pain in chest, oedema, fever, impotence and sterility.

Oil massage, tub bath and enemas are useful. The diet should contain predominantly rice, milk, chicken, milk medicated with *kapikacchu* seeds, *panchamula*, *gokshura* and cucumber seeds. The patient should have sexual intercourse with attractive women.

Suppression of Tears : One sheds tears out of joy or sorrow. Suppression of tears results in pain in the eyes, diseases of eyes, headache, heaviness in head, giddiness and neck stiffness. If chronic, suppression can lead to anorexia, cold, sinusitis, heart disease and cystic swelling in the eyelid.

The treatment consists of inducing tear secretion or inducing sleep by telling pleasant stories. Taking medicated oil or ghee and induction of sweating are also useful.

Suppression of Hunger : Suppression of hunger gives rise to hunger, anorexia, weakness, emaciation, discoloration of skin, bodyache, pain in chest, exhaustion, giddiness, diminished acuity of vision and drowsiness.

The treatment consists of taking small quantities of light, unctuous and warm diet frequently,

Suppression of Thirst : Suppression of thirst gives rise to dryness of mouth and throat, dehydration, exhaustion, pain in chest, difficulty in hearing, deafness, giddiness and drowsiness.

The treatment consists of giving cold drinks and bath with cold water. *Mantha,* i.e. *satu* in adequate quantity together with ghee should be soaked in cold water so as to give it a semi-solid consistency and should be given frequently. *Yavagu,* i.e. thin rice *kanji* prepared by adding six times more water should be administered frequently.

Suppression of Sleep : Suppression of sleep gives rise to yawning, laziness, heaviness of eyes, head and body, bodyache, headache and drowsiness. The treatment consists of inducing sleep by drinking buffalo's milk or fresh (unboiled) cow's milk, light massage and listening to pleasant stories. In addition to the above biological urges mentioned in the literature, it is important to respect and not to suppress any urge, e.g. urge to maintain optimum body temperature. Thus, when one feels chilly, one should not suppress the desire for warm clothes, warm room and hot food and vice-versa.

COMPLICATIONS, SEQUELE, PROGNOSIS AND TREATMENT

Complications and Sequele : Suppression or induction of urges can give rise to any disease predominantly of *Vataja* variety.

Prognosis : Excessive thirst, severe colicky pain, vomiting of faceal matter and emaciation indicate bad prognogis in patients suffering from diseases due to suppression of biological urges.

Treatment : The treatment is directed towards educating the patient to attend promptly to, and never to suppress the biological urges. *Vataprakopa* is the end result of suppression of all the urges. Hence, one should advise diet, activities and medicines which would subdue and normalise the increased *Vata*. In addition suppression of some biological urges result in accumulation of waste products, which can be dangerous to life. Hence, one should always be vigilant and see that the waste products do not accumulate in the body, e.g. frequent micturition is advised for evacuation of residual urine in bladder atony. One should use enemas, purgatives, emetics and snuffs, etc. to see that the wast products do not collcct and are not retained in the body.

As opposed to biological urges related to biological needs which should never be suppressed, one should always exert and control all other desire instincts, emotions and mental processes. Thus, one should always attempt control one's sex instinct, though once involved in the sex act one should not suppress ejaculation. Similarly, one should control one's sorrow, though one should not try to suppress tears. One should always exercise control over one's, emotions like fear, anger, envy, jealousy, hatred, greed and love in excess. One should always suppress impulses to steal and to harm others and behave shamelessly. One should always inhibit impulses to make harsh, untimely or false statements while speaking. One should continuously exercise control over one's sense and motor organs and follow the dictates of his conscience. One should always follow the rules of good conduct and while following these, should not get attached to the worldly affairs. Thus, a person who controls his mental processes enjoys a happy and healthy life.

वेगावरोध:

न वेगान् धारयेद् धमाञ्जातान् मूत्रपुरीषयो:।

न रेतसो न वातस्य नच्छर्द्या: क्षवथोर्न च।

नोद्गरस्य न जृम्भाया न वेगान् क्षुत्पिपासयो:।

न वाष्पस्य न निद्राया नि:श्वासस्य श्रमेण च।।   (च. सू. 7/3-4)

अधश्चोद्ध्वंञ्च भावानां प्रवृत्तानां स्वभावत:।

न वेगान् धारयेत् प्राज्ञो वातादीनां जिजीविषु:।।

वाताविण्मूत्रजृम्भाश्रुक्षवथूद्गारवमीन्द्रियै:।

व्याहन्यमानैरुदितैरुदावर्त्तो निरुच्यते।।

क्षुत्तृष्णाश्वासनिद्राणामुदावर्त्तो विधारणात्।

तस्याभिधास्ये व्यासेन लक्षणञ्च चिकित्सितम्।।   (सु. उ. 55/3-5)

वेगान्नधारयेद्वातविण्मूत्रक्षवतृट्क्षुधाम्।

निद्राकासश्रमश्वासजृम्भाश्रुच्छदिरेरितसाम्।।   (अ. हृ. सू. 4/1)

वेगरोधाद्वातप्रकोप:

रोगा: सर्वेऽपि जायन्ते वेगोदीरणधारणै:।

निर्निष्टं साधनं तत्र भूयिष्ठं ये तु तान् प्रति।।

ततश्चानेकधा प्राय: पवनो यत्रकुप्यति।

अन्नपानौषधं तस्य युञ्जीतातोऽनुलोमनम्।।   (अ. हृ. सू. 4/22-23)

वेगोधारणम् वेगोदीरणम् च

यद्यपि वेगोदीरणधारणात्सर्वे रोगा जायन्ते इत्युक्तम्। तथापि यथा वेगधारणाच्चि-रकालभाविन: सप्रत्यया रोगा भवन्ति न तथोदीरणात्। अतएव तन्त्रकारोऽधावातस्य रोधेनापि रोगा भवन्ति। शकृतो रोधादमी भक्तीन्त्युवाच। न तु तदुदीरणादमी रोगा भवन्तीति।

(सर्वाङ्गिसुन्दरटीका (अरुणदत्त) श्लो. 24, अ. हृ. सू. 4)

वेगधारणम्

अपान वायु:

सङ्गो विण्मूत्रवातानामाध्मानं वेदना क्लम:।

जठरे वातजाश्चान्ये रोगा: स्युर्वातनिग्रहात्।। (च. सू. 7/12)

आध्मानशूलौ हृदयोपरोधं शिरोरुजं श्वासमतीव हिक्काम्।

कासप्रतिश्यायगलग्रहांश्च बलासपित्तप्रसरश्च घोरम्।।

कुर्यादपानोऽभिहत: स्वमार्गे हन्यात् पुरीषं मुखत: क्षिपेद्वा।। (सु. उ. 55/17)

अधोवातस्य रोधेन गुल्मोदावर्तरुकक्लमा:।

वातमूत्रशकृत्सङ्गदृष्ट्याग्निवधहृद्गदा:।। (अ. हृ. सू. 4/12)

चिकित्सा

स्नेहस्वेदविधिस्तत्र वर्तयो भोजनानि च।

पानानि बस्तयश्चैतव शस्तं वातानुलोमनम्।। (च. सू. 7/13)

आस्थापनं मारुतजे स्निग्धस्विन्ने विशिष्यते।

पुरीषजे तु कर्तव्यो विविधरानाहिको भवेत्।। (सु. उ. अ. 55/20)

पुरीष वेगावरोध:

पक्वाशयशिर:शूलं वातवर्चोऽप्रवर्तनम्।

पिण्डिकोद्वेष्ठनाध्मानं पुरीषे स्याद् विधारिते।। (च. सू. 7/8)

आटोपशूलौ परिकर्त्तनञ्च सङ्ग्रहपुरीषस्य तथोद्ध्वता:।

पुरीषमास्यादपि वा निरेति पुरीषवेगेऽभिहते नरस्य।। (सु. उ. 55/8)

शकृत: पिण्डिकोद्वेष्टप्रतिश्यायशिरोरुज:।

ऊर्ध्ववायु: परीकर्तो हृदयस्योपरोधनम्।। (अ. हृ. सू. 4/4)

मुखेन विट्प्रवृत्तिश्च पूर्वोक्तामया: स्मृता।।

तृष्णार्दितं परिक्लिष्टं क्षीणं शूलैरभिद्रुतम्।

शकृद्वमन्तं मतिमानुदावर्तिनमुत्सृजेत्।। (अ. सं. उ. 55/5, 38)

चिकित्सा

स्वेदाभ्यङ्गावगाहाश्च वर्तयो वस्तिकर्म च।

हितं प्रतिहते वर्चस्यन्नपानं प्रमाथि च।। (च. सू. 7/9)

वर्त्यभ्यङ्गावगाहाश्च स्वेदं वस्तिकर्म च।।

अन्नपानं च विड्भेदी विड्रोधोत्थेषु यक्ष्मसु।   (अ. हृ. सू. 4/6, 20)

पुरीषजे तु कर्त्तव्यो विधिरानाहिको भवेत्।।   (सु. उ. 55/20)

आनाहमामप्रभवं जयेत् तु प्रच्छर्दनैर्लङ्घनपाचनैश्च।   (च. चि. 26)

आमोद्भवे वान्तमुपक्रमेत संसर्गभक्तक्रम दीपनीयै:।

अथैतरंयो न शकृद्वमेत्तमामज्ञयेत् स्वेदन पाचनै: च।।   (सु. उ. 57/23)

मूत्रवेगावरोध:

बस्तिर्मेहनयो: शूलं मूत्रकृच्छ्रं शिरोरुजा।

विनामो वंक्षणानाह: स्याल्लिङ्गं मूत्र निग्रहे।।

मूत्रस्य वेगेऽभिहते नरस्तु कृच्छ्रेण मूत्रं कुरुतेऽल्पमल्पम्।।

मेढ्रे गुदे वङ्क्षणबस्तिमुष्कनाभिप्रदेशेष्वथवाऽपि मूर्ध्नि।

आनाद्धबस्तिश्च भवन्ति तीव्रा: शूलाश्च शूलैरिव भिन्नमूर्ते:।।

                                                        (सु. उ. 55/19-10)

अङ्गभङ्गाश्मरीवस्ति मेढ्रवङ्क्षणवेदना:।

मूत्रस्य रोधात्पूर्वे च प्रायो रोगा: भवन्ति हि।।   (अ. हृ. सू. 4/5)

चिकित्सा

स्वेदावगाहनाभ्यङ्गान् सर्पिजषश्चावपीडकम्।

मूत्रे प्रतिहते कुर्यात् त्रिविधं बस्तिकर्म च।।   (च. सू. 7/7)

वर्त्यम्भङ्गावगाहाश्च स्वेदनं वस्तिकर्म च।।

मूत्रजेषु च पाने च प्राग्भक्तं शस्यते घृतम्।

जीर्णान्तिकं चोत्तमया मात्रया योजनाद्वयम्।।

अवपींडकमेतश्च संज्ञितम्।   (अ. ह. सू. 4/6-7)

सौवर्चलाढ्यां मदिरां मूत्रेत्वभिहते पिबेत्।

एलां वाऽप्यभ मद्येन क्षीरं वाऽपि पिबेन्नर:।।

धात्री फलानां स्वरसं सजलं वा पिबेत् त्र्यहं।

रसं अश्वपुरीषस्य गर्दभस्याऽथवा पिबेत्।।

मासोपदंशं मधु वा पिबेत् वा सीधु गौडिकं।

भद्रादारु वनं मूर्वा हरिद्रा मधुकं तथा।।

कोलप्रमाणानि पिबेत् अन्तरिक्षेण वारिणा।

दु:स्पर्शा स्वरसं वाऽपि कषायं कुङ्कमस्य च।।

एर्वारुबीजं तोयेन पिबेत्वाऽलवणीकृतम्।।

पञ्चमूली श्रुतं क्षीरं द्राक्षारसमथापि वा।

योगांश्च वितरेदत्र पूर्वोक्तानश्मरीदिदः।।

मूत्रकृच्छ्रक्लमं चापि कुर्यात् निखशेषतः।

भूयो वक्ष्यामि योगान् तान् मूत्राधातोपशान्तये।।

वमनवेगावरोधः

कण्डूकोठारुचिव्यङ्गशोथपाण्ड्वामयज्वराः।

कुष्ठहृल्लासवीसर्पाश्छर्दिनिग्रहजा गदाः।।   (च. सू. अ. 7/4)

छर्दिर्विघातेन भवेच्च कुष्ठं येनैव दोषेण विदग्धमन्नम्।।   (सु. उ. 55/14)

विसर्पकोठकुष्ठाक्षिकण्डूपाण्ड्वामयज्वराः।

सकासश्वासहृल्लासःव्यङ्गश्वथवो वमेः।।   (अ. हृ. सू. 4/17)

चिकित्सा

भुक्त्वा प्रच्छर्दनं धूमो लङ्घनं रक्तमोक्षणम्।

रुक्षान्नपानं व्यायामो विरेकश्चान शस्यते।।   (च. सू. 7/15)

छद्यांघातं यदादोषं सम्यक् स्नेहादिभिर्जयेत्।

सक्षारलवणोपेतमभ्यङ्गं चात्रदापयेत्।।

गण्डूषधूमानाहारा रुक्षं भुक्त्वा तदुद्धमः।

व्यायामः सुतिरस्वस्य शस्तं चात्र विरेचनम्।।

सक्षारलवणं तैलमभ्यङ्गार्थं च शस्यते।।   (अ. हृ. सू. 4/18-20)

कासवेग धारणम्

कास्य रोधात्तद्वृद्धिः श्वासारुचिहृदामयाः।

शोषो हिध्मा च।।   (अ. सं. सू. 5/17)

चिकित्सा

कार्योऽत्र कासहा सुतरां विधिः।।   (अ. सं. सू. 5/17)

श्रमश्वास वेगावरोधः

गुल्महृद्रोगसम्मोहाः श्रमानिःश्वासधारणात् जायन्ते।   (च. सू. 7/24)

श्रान्तस्य निःश्वासविनिग्रहेण हृद्रोगमोहावथवाऽपि गुल्मः।।

(सु. उ. 55/17)

गुल्महृद्रोगसम्मोहः श्रमश्वासद्विधारितात्।।   (अ. हृ. सू. 4/14)

चिकित्सा

तत्र विश्रामो वातघ्नश्च क्रिया हिताः।।   (च. सू. 7/24)

भोज्यो रसेन विश्रान्तः श्रमश्वासातुरो नरः।।   (सु. उ. 55/35)

हितं विश्रमणं तत्र वातघ्नश्च क्रियाक्रमः।।   (अ. हृ. सू. 4/15)

क्षवथु वेगावरोधः

मन्यास्तम्भः शिरःशूलमार्दिताधार्धवभेदकौ।

इन्द्रियाणां च दौर्बल्यं क्षवथोः स्याद्विधारणात्।।   (च. सू. 7/16)

भवन्ति गाढं क्षवथोर्विघाताच्छिरोऽक्षिनासाश्रवणेषु रोगा।

कण्ठस्यपूर्णत्वमतीव तोदः।

कूजश्च वायोरुत वाऽप्रवृत्तिः।।   (सु. उ. 55/13)

शिरोर्तीन्द्रियदौर्बल्यमन्यास्तम्भादितं क्षुते।।   (अ. हृ. सू. 4/10)

तत्रोर्ध्वजत्रुकेऽभ्यङ्गः स्वेदो धूमः सनावनः।

हितं वातघ्नमाद्यं च घृतं चोत्तरभक्तिकम्।।   (च. सू. 7/17)

तीक्ष्णाञ्जनावपीडाभ्यां तीक्ष्ण गन्धोपशिङ्घनैः।

वर्तिप्रयोगैरथवा क्षवसंक्तिं प्रवर्तयेत्।।   (सु. उ. 55/29)

तीक्ष्णौषधपधमनैरथवाऽऽदित्यरश्मिभिः।।

तीक्ष्णधूमाञ्जनाघ्राणनावनार्कविलोकनैः।

प्रवर्तयेत्क्षुतिं सक्तां स्नेहस्वेदौ च शीलयेत्।।   (अ. हृ. सू. 4/10)

जृम्भावेगधारणम्

विनामाक्षेपसङ्क्रोचाः सुप्तिः कम्पः प्रवेपनम् जृम्भाया निग्रहः।।

                                                            (च. सू. 7/19)

मन्यागलस्तम्भशिरोविकारा।

जृम्भोपघातात् पनात्मका स्युः।

श्रोत्राननघ्राणविलोचनोत्था।

भवन्ति तीव्राश्च तथा विकाराः।।   (सु. उ. 55/11)

जृम्भाया: क्षववद्रोगा: सर्वश्चानिलनिग्रिधः।।   (अ. हृ. सू. 54/16)

शिरोऽत्तीन्द्रियदौर्बल्यमन्यास्तम्भार्दितं क्षुते।।   (अ. हृ. सू. 4/10)

चिकित्सा

तत्र सर्वं वातघ्नमौषधम्।। (च. सू. 7/19)

स्नेहै: स्वेदैरुदावर्त्तं जृम्भाजं समुपाचरेत्।

अश्रुमोक्षोऽश्रुजे कार्य: स्निग्धस्विन्नस्य देहिन:।। (सु. उ. 55/28)

सर्वश्च अनिल जित् विधि:।। (अ. ह्. सू. 4/16)

उद्गारवेगोधारणम्

हिक्का: श्वासोऽरुचि: कम्पो विबन्धो हृदयोरसो:।

उद्गार निग्रहात् तत्र हिक्कायास्तुल्यमौषधम्।। (च. सू. 7/18)

कण्ठास्यपूर्णत्वमतीव तोद:।

कूजश्च वायोरुत वाऽप्रवृत्ति:।।

उद्गारवेगेऽभिहते भवन्ति।

घोरा विकारा: पवनप्रसूता:।। (सु. उ. 55/13-14)

उद्गारस्यारुचि: कम्पो विबन्धो हृदयोरसो:।

आध्मानकासहिध्माश्चहिध्मावत्तत्रभेषजम्। (अ. सं. सू. 5)

चिकित्सा

तत्र हिक्कायास्तुल्यमौषधम्।। (च. सू. 7/18)

उद्गारजे क्रमोपेतं स्नैहिकं धूममाचरेत्।

सुरां सौवर्चलवर्तीं बीजपूरसान्वितम्।। (सु. उ. 55/130)

कार्योऽत्र कासहा सुतरां विधि:।। (अ. ह्. सू. 4/14)

वाष्पवेगावरोध:

प्रतिश्यायोऽक्षिरोगश्च हृद्रोगश्चारुचिभ्रम: बाष्पनिग्रहणात्।।

(च. सू. 7/22)

आनन्दजं शोकसमुद्भवं वा नेत्रोदकं प्राप्तममुञ्चतो हि।

शिरोगुरुत्वं नयनामयाश्च भवन्ति तीव्रा: सह पीनसेन।। (सु. उ. 55/12)

पीनसाक्षि शिरोहृद्ङ्मन्यस्तम्भारुचिभ्रमा:।

सगुल्मा बाष्पत:।। (अ. ह्. सू. 4/17)

चिकित्सा

तत्र स्वप्नो मद्यं प्रिया: कथा:।। (च. सू. 7/22)

अश्रुमोक्षोऽश्रुजे कार्य: स्निग्धस्विन्नस्य देहिन:।।   (सु. उ. 55/28)

क्षुधावेगधारणम्

कार्श्यदौर्बल्यवैवर्णमङ्गमर्दोऽरुचिभ्रम:।

क्षुद्धेगनिग्राहात् तत्र स्निग्धोष्णं लघुभोजनम्।।   (च. सू. 7/20)

तन्द्राऽङ्गमर्दावरुचिभ्रमा: स्यु:क्षुधोभिघातात् कृशता च दृष्टे:।

कण्ठास्यशोष: श्रवणावरोध तृष्णाभिघाताद् हृदये व्यथा च।।

(सु. उ. 55/16)

अङ्गभङ्गारुचिग्लानिकार्श्यशूलभ्रमा: क्षुध:।।   (अ. हृ. सू. 4/12)

चिकित्सा

तत्र स्निग्धोष्णं लघु भोजनं।।   (च. सू. 7/20)

क्षुद्विघाते हितं स्निग्धमुष्णमल्पञ्च भोजनम्।।   (सु. उ. 55/34)

तत्र योज्यं लघु स्निग्धमुष्णल्पं च भोजनम्।।   (अ. हृ. सू. 4/12)

पिपासा वेगधारणम्

कण्ठास्यशोषो बाधिर्य श्रम: सादो हृदि व्यथा पिपासा निग्रहात्।।

(च. सू. 7/21)

कण्ठास्यशोष: श्रवणावरोध स्तृष्णाऽभिघाताद् हृदये व्यथा च।।

(सु. उ. 55/16)

शोषङ्गसादबाधिर्यसम्मोहभ्रमहृद्गदा:।

तृष्णाया निग्रहात्।   (अ. हृ. सू. 4)

चिकित्सा

तत्र शीतं तर्पणमिष्यते।।   (च. सू. 7/21)

तृष्णाघाते पिबेन्मथ यवागूं वाऽपि शीतलाम्।।   (सु. उ. 55/34)

तत्र शीत: सर्वो विधिहितं।।   (अ. हृ. सू. 4/11)

निद्रावेगधारणम्

जृम्भाऽङ्गमर्दस्तन्द्रा च शिरोरोगोऽक्षिगौरवम्।

निद्राविधारणात्।।   (च. सू. 7/23)

जृम्भाऽङ्गमर्दोऽङ्ग शिरोऽभिक्षजाड्यं।

निद्राऽभिघातादथवाऽपि तन्द्रा।।   (सु. उ. 55/17)

निद्राया मोहमूर्धाक्षिगौरवालस्यजृम्भिका:।।

अङ्गमर्द: च। (अ. हृ. सू. 4/13)

चिकित्सा

तत्र स्वप्नं संवाहनानि च।। (च. सू. 7/23)

निद्राघाते पिबेत् क्षीरं स्वप्याच्चेष्टकथा नर:।। (सु. उ. 55/35)

तत्र इष्ट: स्वप्न: संवाहनानि च।। (अ. हृ. सू. 4/13)

वेगोधारणे उपद्रवा:

रोगा: सर्वेऽपि जायन्ते वेगोदीरणधारणै:।। (अ. हृ. सू. 4/23)

एतान् धारयतो जातान् वेगान् रोगा भवन्ति।। (च. सू. 7/23)

वेगोधारणे साध्यासाध्यत्वम्

तृदशूलार्त्तं त्यजेत्क्षीणं विड्वमं वेगरोधिनम्।। (अ. सं. सू. 5)

धारणीया वेगा:

धारयेत्तु सदा वेगान् हितैषी प्रेत्य चेह च।

लोभेर्ष्याद्वेषमात्सर्यरागादीनां जितेन्द्रिय:।। (अ. हृ. सू. 4/25)

इमांस्तु धारयेद् वेगान् हितार्थी प्रेत्य चेह च।

साहसानामशस्तानां मनोवाक्कायकर्मणाम्।।

लोभशोकभयक्रोधमानवेगान् विधारयेत्।

नैर्लज्ज्येर्ष्यातिरागाणामभिध्यायाँश्च बुद्धिमान्।।

परुषस्यातिमात्रस्य सूचकस्यानृतस्य च।

वाक्यस्याकालयुक्तस्य धारयेद् वेगमुत्थितम्।।

देहप्रवृत्तिर्या काचिद् विद्यते परपीड्या।

स्त्रीभोगस्तेयहिंसाद्या तस्या वेगान् विधारयेत्।।

पुण्यशब्दो विपापत्वामनोवाक्कायकर्मणाम्।

धर्मार्थकामान् पुरुष: सुखी भुङ्क्ते चिनोति च।। (अ. हृ. सू. 4/25-30)

शुक्रवेगावरोध:

मेढ्रे वृषणयो: शूलमङ्गमर्दो हृदि व्यथा।

भवेत् प्रतिहते शुक्रे विबद्धं मूत्रमेव च।। (च. सू. 7/10)

मूत्रोशये पायुनिममुष्कयोश्च।

शोफो रुजो मूत्रविनिग्रहश्च।

शुक्राश्मरी तत्स्ववर्णं भवेद्वा।

ते ते विकारा विहते तु शुक्रे।।   (सु. उ. 55/15)

शुक्रात्तात्स्ववर्णं गुह्यवेदनाश्वयथुज्वरः।

हृद्व्यथामूत्रसङ्गाङ्गभङ्गवृद्धशमषण्ढताः।।   (अ. हृ. सू. 4/20)

चिकित्सा

तत्राभ्यङ्गोऽवगाहश्च मदिरा चरणायुधाः।

शालिः पयो निरुहश्च शस्तं मैथुनमेव च।।   (च. सू. 7/11)

बस्तिशुद्धिकरावापं चतुर्गुणजलं पयः।।

आवारिनाशात् क्वथितं पीतवन्तं प्रकामतः।।

रसयेयुः प्रिया नार्यः शुक्रोदावर्त्तिनं नरम्।।   (सु. उ. 55/32-33)

ताम्रचूडसुराशालिवत्स्यभ्यङ्गावगाहनम्।

बस्तिशुद्धिकरैः सिद्धं भजेत्क्षीरं प्रियाः स्त्रियः।।   (अ. हृ. सू. 4/23)

5

VITIATION OF BODY CHANNELS
(SROTODUSHTI)

WHAT IS SROTAS ?

The word *Srotas* means body passages or body channels. Any body passage or channel, which carries solids, liquids, gases, nerve impulses, nutrients, waste products and secretions from the glands is termed as *srotas*. They held in the circulation of body fluids as well as body elements. Suhruta defines *srotas* as a channel or a passage, which starts from some space in the body and which secretes or carries fluids. These channels do not include blood vessels and nerves. Unlike Sushruta, Charaka defines *srotas* as any natural space or passage in the body and includes blood vessels, i.e. arteries, veins, capillaries, nerves, lymphatics and cavities in the body like stomach, intestine etc. Alternatively, he also defines *srotas* as, "a passage which secretes or from which oozes body fluids". This definition is more applicable to small passages or channels of secreting glands or capillaries and lymphatics.

Some physicians consider that man is nothing but a network of multitude of channels, i.e. *srotas*. The colour of the minute channels is, in general, same as that of the tissues or organs from which they arise.

The body channels are classified as internal channels and channels having their natural orifices on the surface of the body. The two ears, the two eyes, the two nostrils, the mouth, the anus and the urethra are the nine orifices of the body passages opening externally. Females having three more orifices, those of two breasts and the vagina. The internal body channels are divided into large and small channels. The large channels can be counted, while the small channels are innumerable and minute. The intracellular channels are ultramicroscopic and are responsible for carrying nutrients and waste products within the cells. For each new substance secreted or syntbesised by the body there is specific variety of channel. Thus, there are innumerable varieties of channels in the body.

Charaka describes fourteen types of *srotras* while Sushruta describes only eleven types. Sushruta does not include channels of bony tissue, nervous, tissue and sweat glands in *srotas*. The *doshas*, viz. *Vata*, *Pitta* and *Kapha* do not have special channels of their own, as they have free access to all the body tissues and channels. Charaka being a physician describes the manifestations of vitiation, i.e. the diseased states of various channels, while Sushruta being a surgeon describes the manifestations of injury to the channels.

Vata, *Pitta* and *Kapha* the three *doshas* are responsible for affection of various body channels. The diet and activities having qualities similar to one or more *doshas*, but opposite to that of the affected tissues affect the body channels. Thus, increased *doshas* and the weakened or vitiated tissues, lead to diseases of various channels. The various channels may be injured by accident or during surgery.

SYMPTOMS IN GENERAL

(1) Increased or decreased secretion or flow, e.g. diarrhoea or constipation, polyuria or oliguria, excessive or decreased sweating.

(2) Obstruction to the passage leading to flow in abnormal or reverse direction, e.g. obstructive jaundice, renal calculi, etc.

(3) Hypertrophy or varicosities of vessels, e.g. obstruction to the various channels or body passages is one of the important cause of diseases.

The aetiology, clinical manifestations and line of treatment of vitiation of body channels are described below :

Prana Vaha Srotas : The word *Prana vaha srotas* means channels carrying oxygen. These channels are classified as blood vessels originating from the heart and respiratory passages. These channels get vitiated as a result of wasting, suppression of natural urges, dehydration, undertaking exercise while hungry, starvation and violation of the laws of health. Diseases of these channels result in forceful, restricted, too long or too short, deep or shallow, stertorous and painful respiration. Injuries to these vessels results in groaning, bending down of the body, loss of consciousness, illusion, shivering and ultimately death.

The medical treatment should be on the lines similar to that of *shvasa*, i.e. breathlessness. In case of injury, the appropriate surgical treatment has to be carried out.

Annavaha Srotas : The word *Anna vaha srotas* means channels carrying food. These are represented mainly by gastro-intestinal tract and mesenteric blood vessels carrying nutrients. These channels get vitiated as a result of over-eating, eating at irregular intervals, eating of unwholesome meals and impaired digestive power.

During diseases of these channels, one suffers from disinclination to eat food, anorexia, indigestion, nausea and vomiting. Injury to these channels gives rise to distension, colicky pain, aversion to food, vomiting, thirst, blindness and even death at the end.

The treatment consists of medicines as prescribed for *ama dosha*, i.e. medicines stimulating digestive power and digestion.

Udaka Vaha Srotas : *Udaka vaha srotas* means channels carrying water. These channels consists of palate, pharynx and cloma. Different authorities consider cloma to be adrenal, pancreas or kidney.

These channels are vitiated as a result of heat, indigestion, fright, excessive drinking of alcohol, eating of very dry foods and excessive thirst.

Their pathological states gives rise to dryness of tongue,

palate, lips and throat and intense thirst. Injury to these channels makes the patient thirsty and ultimately results in death.

The case is to be treated on the lines of treatment of the disease *trishna,* i.e. thirst.

Rasa Vaha Srotas : *Rasa vaha srotas,* i.e. channels carrying body fluids. Blood vessels and lymphatics constitute the channels of body fluids. These channels of body fluids get vitiated as a result of worrying too much and eating heavy, cold and oily substances in excessive quantity.

Disinclination for food, anorexia, nausea, impaired sensation of taste, heaviness, fever with bodyache, loss of digestive power, premature wrinkling of the skin and graying of hair are the manifestations of vitiation of these channels. Injury to these channels gives rise to wasting, fainting, shivering, unconsciousness and death.

Fasting is the main line of treatment.

Rakta Vaha Srotas : *Rakta vaha srotas,* i.e. channels carrying blood. Liver and spleen are the main sites of these channels, as these organs store blood and pump it into circulation whenever necessary.

These channels get vitiated by the following factors :

(i) The use of concentrated and hot wines or similar intoxicants.

(ii) The excessive use of salts and alkalies, acids and pungent articles.

(iii) The use of horse-gram, black-gram, *tila* and *tila* oil, common yam, radish etc.

(iv) All varieties of leafy vegetables.

(v) The use of flesh of aquatic animals.

(vi) The use of curd, sour *kanji*, whey, vinegar and *souviraka* wines.

(vii) The use of articles that are incompatible or which have gone soft or are bad smelling.

(viii) Sleeping in the day after having eaten liquid, unctuous and heavy foods.

(ix) Indulgence in over-eating.

(x) Anger and grief.

(xi) Exposure to heat of the Sun and fire.

(xii) Suppression of urge of vomiting.

(xiii) Not practising blood letting at proper season.

(xiv) Fatigue, injury.

(xv) Eating food before previous meal is digested, indigestion and eating on a loaded stomach.

(xvi) The natural tendency of autumn season.

Skin diseases, acutely spreading diseases, menorrhagia, inflammation of rectum, penis and mouth, splenomegaly, gulma, abscesses, bluish-black mole, jaundice, ring-worm, leucoderma, papules, wheals and reddish circular patches arise secondary to affections of these passages.

Injury to these channels results in pallor, cyanosis, fever, burning sensation, haemorrhage and redness of eyes.

The treatment as given in blood disorders, i.e. *rakta pitta* should given.

Mansa Vaha Srotas : The word *Mansa vaha srotas* means channels carrying nutrients to the muscular tissue. These are represented by blood vessels, lymphatics and nerves supplying muscles. These channels are vitiated by sleeping during the day after meal and by consuming large quantities of heavy food items over a long time.

Diseases of these channels gives rise to granuloma, malignant tumors, piles, warts, sloughing of muscles and dry gangrene. Injury to these channels is characterised by swelling, atrophy of muscles, appearance of varicose veins and ultimately death.

The treatment consists of body purification by *panchakarma*, operative measures and cauterisation.

Meda Vaha Srotas : The word *Meda vaha srotas* means channels carrying fat. These channels are represented by intestinal lymphatic ducts. These channels are affected as a result of lack of exercise, sleeping in the day and excessive consumption of fats and wines.

The manifestations of affection of these channels are similar to premonitory signs and symptoms of *prameha*. These are excessive collection of tartar on the teeth, palate and tongue, burning sensation in hands and feet, sticky sweating, thirst and breathlessness. Injury to these channels results in oily perspiration, glossy skin, parched palate, local swelling and thirst.

Treatment as described in obesity should be followed :

Ashthi Vaha Srotas : The word *Asthi vaha srotas* means channels carrying nutrients to bones. Nutrient vessels of the bones constitute these channels, which are usually embedded in fat. These channels are affected as a result of severe exercise, injury to bones, violent body movements and indulgence in other *Vata* promoting activities and dietary factors. Hypertrophy of the bones and teeth, atrophy and pain in the teeth and bones, discolouration and pathological conditions of the hair of the head, body, face and nails are the diseases arising from the morbidity in the bones.

Treatment consists of appropriate *panchakarma* like enemas and administration of milk and ghee medicated with bitter drugs.

Majja Vaha Srotas : The word *Majja vaha srotas* means channels carrying nutrients to nervous tissue, bone-marrow and nerves. These channels are vitiated in crush injuries and compression of bones and indulgence in incompatible food items. Pain in joints, giddiness, fainting and deep seated wound in the joints are the symptoms of diseases of these channels.

The treatment consists of diet and medicines with predominantly sweet and bitter tastes, exercise, administration of emetics in spring and purgatives in autumn.

Shukra Vaha Srotas : The word *Shukra vaha srotas* means channels carrying semen. These channels arise from testes and ducts carrying semen (Seminal vesicles and vas deferens) and open in the urethra.

These channels carrying the semen get vitiated as a result of untimely coitus, unnatural sexual acts, suppression of sexual urge, excessive indulgence in sexual act and from the effects of surgical instruments, alkalies and heat. Affection of these channels result in impotence, sterility, abortion and congenital deformities. Injury to these channels leads to delayed or absence of emission or emission of blood streaked semen.

The treatment consists of diet and medicines predominantly sweet and bitter in taste, exercise, administration of emetics in spring and purgatives is autumn. Intercourse at appropriate interval is beneficial.

Purisha Vaha Srotas : The word *Purisha vaha srotas* means channels carrying faecal matter in colon and rectum. These passages consists of colon and rectum. These channels are vitiated by suppression of urge of defaecation, wasting diseases, weak digestive power, eating in excess and indigestion.

The clinical manifestations of the diseases of these channels are tenesmus with scanty stool, watery or scybalous stools and scanty or copious stools. Injury to these channels is characterised by retention of stools, distension of abdomen and abdominal lump.

The treatment should be advised on the line of diarrhoea or constipation depending on the case.

Mutra Vaha Srotas : The word *Mutra vaha srotas* means the channels carrying urine. These channels include kidney, ureters, bladder and urethra. These channels are vitiated from drinking excessive water and indulging in excess of food and sex, suppressing micturition, wasting diseases and injury to the urinary passages.

Diseases of these channels lead to excessive, interrupted, provoked, scanty or painful micturition. The urine may be thick and may dribble intermittently or continuously. Injury to these passages leads to retention of urine, haemorrhage in bladder and numbness of the genitals.

The treatment as given for the disease dysuria should be administered.

Sveda Vaha Srotas : The word *Sveda vaha srotas* means channels carrying sweat. These channels are vitiated by severe exercise, exposure to heat, indiscriminate indulgence in cold and heat as well as from anger, weeping and fear. Anhidrosis, hyperhidrosis, roughness or excessive smoothness of skin, goose skin and burning sensation are the manifestations of affection of these channels.

The treatment as advised for *Jvara* should be followed.

Artava Vaha Srotas : The word *Artava vaha srotas* means channels of reproductive organs in females, i.e. uterus, fallopian tubes and vagina. Injury to these channels lead to sterility, suppression of menstruation and inability for copulation. The treatment consists of treating the appropriate gynaecological disorder.

GENERAL TREATMENT OF DISEASES OF BODY CHANNELS

The treatment of diseases ese channels consists of administration of diet and pursuing activities, which will subdue the increased *doshas* and strengthen the weakness of the diseased tissues.

In diseases due to obstruction of channels, one should see that the opening of the body channels are kept patent, so that the *doshas* can be easily brought from tissues and organs to the gastro-intestinal tract. Once, they are brought to the gastro-intestinal tract, they can be got rid off by emetics, purgatives or enemas.

स्रोतांसि

सुश्रुतोक्त व्याख्या

मूलात् खादन्तरं देहे प्रसृतं त्वभिवाहि यत्।
स्रोतस्तदिति विज्ञेयं सिराधमनिवर्जितम्।।   (सु. शा. 9/13)

चरकोक्त व्याख्या

सर्वे हि भावाः पुरुषे नान्तरेण स्रोतांस्यभिनिर्वर्तन्ते, क्षयं वाऽप्यभिगच्छन्ति।

स्रोतांसि खलु परिणाममापद्यमानानां धातूनामभिवाहीनि भवन्तिययनार्थेन।।

(च. वि. 5/3)

स्रवणात् स्रोतांसि ।

(च. सू. 30)

स्रवणात् इति रसादे: पोष्यस्यस्रवणात् ।

(चक्रपाणिटीका)

तेषां तु मलप्रसादाख्यानां धातूनां स्रोतांस्ययनमुखानि ।

तानि यथाविभागेन यथास्वं धातूनापूरयन्ति ।।

(च. सू. 28/5)

स्रोतस: स्वरूपम्

स्वधातुसमवर्णानि वृत्तस्थूलान्यणूनि च ।

स्रोतांसिदीर्घाण्याकृत्या प्रतानसदृशानि च ।।

(च. वि. 5/25)

स्रोतसांसंख्या

स्रोतांसिद्विविधानि- बर्हिर्मुखानि अन्तर्मुखानि च ।

तत्र अन्तर्मुखान्येव योगवाहीनि स्रोतांसि ।

श्रवण-नयन-वदन-घ्राण-गुद-मेढ्राणि नव स्रोतांसि नराणां बहिर्मुखानि, एतान्येव स्त्रीणामपराणि च त्रीणि द्वे स्तनयोरधस्ताद्रक्तवहं च ।

(सु. शा. 5/10)

अतिबहुत्वात् खलु केचिदपरिसङ्ख्येयान्याचक्षते स्रोतांसि, परिसङ्ख्येयानि पुनरन्दे ।

(च. वि. 5/5)

यावन्त: पुरुषे मूर्तिमन्तो भावविशेषास्तावन्त एवास्मिन् स्रोतसां प्रकारविशेष: ।

(च. वि. 5/1)

प्राणोदकान्नरसरुधिरमांसमेदोस्थिमज्जशुक्रमूत्रपुरीषस्वेदवहानीति; वातपित्तश्लेष्माणां पुन: सर्वशरीरचराणां सर्वाणि स्रोतांस्ययनभूतानि ।

(आ. श. भा. 2; पृ. 1683 च. वि. 5/6)

शल्यतन्त्रे तु स्रोता स्येकादशैव, तानि पुन: प्राणान्नोदकरसरक्तमांसमेदोमूत्र-पुरीषशुक्रार्तववहानि, येष्वधिकार: शल्यतन्त्रे ।

(सु. शा. 9'12; आ. श. भ. 2; पृ. 1883)

शल्यतन्त्रे तु अस्थिमज्जस्वेदवहानां स्रोतसां नोल्लेख: ।   (डल्हण)

स्रोतसां दुष्टिकारणम्

सामान्येन सर्वेषामेव स्रोतसां वातपित्तश्लेष्माण: प्रदुष्टा दूषयितारो भवन्ति, दोषस्वभावादिति ।

(च. वि. 5/9)

आहारश्च विहारश्च यः स्याद्दोषगुणैः समः धातुभिर्विगुणश्चापि स्रोतसां स प्रदूषकः।

(च. वि. 5/23)

स्रोतोदुष्टिलक्षणानि

अतिप्रवृत्तिः सङ्गो वा सिराणां ग्रन्थयोऽपि वा। विमार्गगमनं चापि स्रोतसां
दुष्टिलक्षणम्।

(च. वि. 5/24)

प्राणवह स्रोतस्

तत्र प्राणवहानां स्रोतसां हृदयं मूलं महास्रोतश्च।   (च. वि. 5/7)

प्राणवहे द्वे तर्योर्मूलं हृदयं रसहवाहिन्यश्च धमन्यः।   (सु. शा. 9)

प्राणवह स्रोतोदुष्टिकारणानि

क्षयात् सन्धारणाद् रौक्ष्याद् व्यायामात् क्षुधितस्य च।
प्राणवाहीनि दुष्यन्ति स्रोतांस्यन्यैश्च दारुणैः।।

(च. वि. 5/10)

प्राणवह स्रोतोदुष्टिलक्षणानि

अतिसृष्टमतिबद्धं कुपितमल्पाल्पभीक्ष्णं वा सशब्दशूलमुच्छ्वसन्तं दृष्ट्वा
प्राणवहान्यस्य स्रोतांसि प्रदुष्यनीति विद्यात्।।

(च. वि. 5/7)

विद्धलक्षणानि

तत्र विद्धस्याक्रोशनविनमन-मोहन-भ्रमण-वेपनाति मरणं वा भवति।

(सु. शा. 9/12)

चिकित्सा

प्राणोदकान्नवाहानां दुष्टानां श्वासिकी क्रिया।
कार्या तृष्णोपशमनी तथैवामप्रदोषिकी।।

(च. वि. 5/26)

अन्नवह स्रोतस्

अन्नवहानां स्रोतसामाशयो मूलं वामं च पार्श्व।   (च. वि. 5/8)

अन्नवहे द्वे तयोर्मूलमामाशयोऽन्नवाहिन्यश्च धमन्यः।   (सु. शा. 9/12)

अन्नवहस्रोतो दुष्टिकारणानि

अतिमात्रस्य चाकाले चाहितस्य च भोजनात्।
अन्नवाहीनि दुष्यन्ति वैगुण्यात् पावकस्य च।।

(च. वि. 5/12)

अन्नवहस्रोतो दुष्टिलक्षणानि

अन्नाभिलक्षणमरोचकविपाकौ छर्दि च दृष्ट्वाऽन्नवहान्यस्य स्रोतांसि प्रदुष्टानिति
विद्यात् । (च. वि. 5/8)

विद्धलक्षणानि

तत्र विद्धस्याध्मानं शूलोऽन्नद्वेषच्छर्दिः पिपासाऽऽन्ध्यं मरणं च ।

(सु. शा. 9/12)

चिकित्सा

प्राणोदकान्नवाहानां दुष्टानां श्वासिकी क्रिया ।
कार्या तृष्णोपशमनी तथैवामप्रदोषिकी । (च. वि. 5/26)

उदकवह स्रोतस्

उदकवहानां स्रोतसां तालुमूलं क्लोम च । (च. वि. 5/8)
उदकवहे द्वे, तयोर्मूलं तालु क्लोम च । (सु. शा. 9/12)

उदकवहस्रोतो दुष्टिकारणानि

औष्ण्यादामाद् भयात् पानादतिशुष्कान्नसेवनात् ।
अम्बुवाहीनि दुष्यन्ति तृष्णायाश्चातिपीडनात् ।। (च. वि. 5/11)

उदकवहस्रोतो दुष्टिलक्षणानि

जिह्वातालुवोष्ठकण्ठक्लोमशोषं पिपासां चातिप्रवृद्धां दृष्ट्वोदकवहान्यस्य स्रोतांसि
प्रदुष्टानिति विधात् । (च. वि. 5/8)

विद्धलक्षणानि

तत्र विद्धस्य पिपासा (पिपासाऽसाध्या श्यावा ङ्गता 'पाठः', सद्योमरणं च ।

(सु. शा. 9/12)

चिकित्सा

प्राणोदकान्नवाहानां दुष्टानां श्वासिकी क्रिया ।
कार्या तृष्णोपशमनी तथैवामप्रदोषिकी ।। (च. वि. 26)

रसवह स्रोतस्

रसवहानां स्रोतसां हृदयं मूलं दश च धमन्यः । (च. वि. 5/8)
रसवहे द्वे, तयोर्मूलं हृदयं रसवाहिन्यश्च धमन्यः ।। (सु. शा. 9/12)

रसवहस्रोतो दुष्टिकारणानि

गुरुशीतमतिस्निग्धमतिमात्रं समशनताम्।
रसवाहीनि दुष्यन्ति चिन्त्यानां चातिचिन्तनात्।   (च. वि. 5/13)

रसवहस्रोतो दुष्टिलक्षणानि

अश्रद्धा चारुचिरास्यवैरस्यमरसज्ञता।
हल्लासो गौरवं तन्द्रा साङ्गमर्दो ज्वरस्तम:।
पाण्डुत्वं स्रोतसां रोध: क्लैव्यं साद: कृशाङ्गता।
नाशोऽग्नेरयथाकालं वलय: पलितानि च।   (च. सू. 28/9, 10)

विद्धलक्षणानि

तत्र विद्धस्य शोष: प्राणवहविद्धवच्च मरणं तल्लिङ्गानि च।   (सु. शा. 9/12)

चिकित्सा

रसजानां विकाराणां सर्वलङ्घनमौषधम्।   (च. सू. 28/25)

रक्तवह स्रोतस्

शोणितवहानां स्रोतसां यकृन्मूलं प्लीहा च।   (च. वि. 5/8)
रक्तवहे द्वे, तयोर्मूलं यकृत्प्लीहानौ रक्तवाहिन्यश्च धमन्य:।   (सु. शा. 9/12)

रक्तवहस्रोतो दुष्टिकारणानि

विदाहीन्यन्नपानानि स्निग्धोष्णानि द्रवाणि च।
रक्तवाहीनि दुष्यन्ति भजतां चातपानलौ।।   (च. वि. 5/14)

प्रदुष्टबहुतीक्ष्णोष्णैर्मद्यैरन्यैश्च तद्विधै:।
तथाऽतिलवणक्षारैरम्लै: कटुभिरेव च।।
कुलत्थमाषनिष्पावतिलतैलनिषेवणै:।
पिण्डालुमूलकादीनां हरितानां च सर्वश:।।
जलजानूपबैलानां प्रसहानां च सेवनात्।
दध्यम्लमस्तुसुक्तानां सुरासौवीरकस्य च।।
विरुद्धानामुपक्लिन्नपूतीनां भक्षणेन च।
भुक्त्वा दिवा प्रस्वपतां द्रवस्निग्धगुरुणि च।।
अत्यादानं तथा क्रोधं भजतां चातपानलौ।
छर्दिवेगप्रतीघातात् काले चानवसेचनात्।।
श्रमाभिघातसन्तापैरजीर्णाध्यशनैस्तथा।
शरत्कालस्वभावाच्च शोणितं सम्प्रदुष्यति।।   (च. सू. 24/5-10)

रक्तवहस्त्रोतो दुष्टिलक्षणानि

कुष्ठविसर्पपिडकारक्तपित्तमसृग्दर:।।
गुदमेढ्रास्यपाकश्च प्लीहा गुल्मोऽथ विद्रधि:।
नीलिका कामला व्यङ्ग: पिल्पवस्तिलकालका:।
ददुश्चर्मदलं श्वित्रं पामा कोठास्त्रमण्डलम् । रक्तप्रदोषाज्जायन्ते।

(च. सू. 28/11,12)

विद्धलक्षणानि

तत्र विद्धस्य श्यावाङ्गता ज्वरो दाह: पाण्डुता शोणितागमनं रक्तनेत्रता च।

(सु. शा. 6/12)

चिकित्सा

विधिशोणितिकेऽध्याये रक्तजानां भिषग्जितम्।   (च. सू. 28/26)
कुर्याच्छोणितरोगेषु रक्तपित्तहरीं क्रियाम्।
विरेकमुपवासं च स्त्रावणं शोणितस्य च।।   (च. सू. 24/18)

मांसवह स्त्रोतस्

मांसवहानां स्त्रोतसां स्नायुमूलं त्वक् च।   (च. वि. 5/8)
मांसवहे द्वे, तयोर्मूलं स्नायुत्वचं रक्तवहाश्च धमन्या।   (सु. शा. 9/12)

मांसवहस्त्रोतो दुष्टिकारणानि

अभिष्यन्दीनि भोज्यानि स्थूलानि च गुरुणि च।
मांसवाहीनि दुष्यन्ति भुक्त्वा व स्वपतां दिवा।।   (च. वि. 5/15)

मांसवहस्त्रोतो दुष्टिलक्षणानि

अधिमांसार्बुदं कीलं गलशालूकशुण्डिके।
पूतिमांसालजीगण्डगण्डमालोपजिह्विका:।
विद्यान्मांसाश्रयान्।   (च. सू. 28/14)

विद्धलक्षणानि

तत्र विद्धस्य श्वयथुमांसशोष: सिराग्रन्थयो मरणं च।   (सु. शा. 9/12)

चिकित्सा

मांसजानां तु संशुद्धि: शस्त्रक्षाराग्निकर्म च।
अष्टौ निन्दितिकेऽध्याये मेदोजानां चिकित्सितम्।   (च. सू. 28/26)

मेदवह स्रोतस्

मेदोवहे द्वे, तयोर्मूलं कटि वृक्कौ च। (सु. शा. 9/12)

मेदोवहानां स्रोतसां वृक्कौ मूलं वपावहनं च। (च. वि. 5/8)

मेदवहस्रोतो दुष्टिकारणानि

अव्यायामाद् दिवास्वप्नान्मेद्यानां चातिभक्षणात्।

मेदोवाहीनि दुष्यन्ति वारुण्याश्चातिसेवनात्।। (च. वि. 5/16)

मेदवहस्रोतो दुष्टिलक्षणानि

मेद: संश्रयांस्तु प्रचक्ष्महे।

निन्दितानि प्रमेहाणां पूर्वरूपाणि यानि च।। (च. सू. 28/15)

दन्तानीनां मलाढ्यत्वं प्रागूपं पाणिपादयो:।

दाहश्चक्कणतादेहे तृट्श्वासश्चोपजायते। (मा. नि. पृ. 142)

विद्धलक्षणानि

तत्र विद्धस्य स्वेदागमनं स्निग्धाङ्गता तालुशोष: स्थूलता शोफ: पिपासा च।

(सु. शा. 9/12)

चिकित्सा

अष्टौ निन्दितिकेऽध्याये मेदोजानां चिकित्सितम्।। (च. सू. 28/27)

सततं व्याधितावेतावतिस्थूलकृशौ नरौ।

सततं चोपचर्यौ हि कर्शणैर्बृंहणैरपि। (च. सू. 21/16)

अस्थिवह स्रोतम्

अस्थिवहानां स्रोतसां मेदो मूलं जघनं च। (च. वि. 5/8)

अथिवहस्रोतो दुष्टिकारणानि

व्यायामदतिसङ्क्षोभादस्थ्नामतिविघट्टनात्।

अस्थिवाहीनि दुष्यन्ति वातलानां च सेवनात्। (च. वि. 5/17)

अस्थिवहस्रोतो दुष्टिलक्षणानि

अध्यस्थिदन्तौ दन्तास्थिभेदशूलं विवर्णता।

क्वेशलोमनखश्मश्रुदोषाश्चास्थिप्रदोषजा:। (च. सू. 28/16)

अध्यस्थ्यधिदन्तास्थितोदशूलकुनरवप्रभृतथोऽस्थिदोषजा:। (सु. सू. 24/14)

चिकित्सा

अस्थ्याश्रयाणां व्याधीनां पञ्चकर्माणि भेषजम्।

बस्तय: क्षीरसर्पींषि तिक्तकोपहितानि च।। (च. सू. 28/27)

मज्जावह स्रोतस्

मज्जवहानां स्रोतसामस्थीनि मूलं सन्धयश्च। (च. वि. 5/8)

मज्जावहस्रोतो दुष्टिकारणानि

उत्पेषदत्यभिष्यन्दादभिघातात् प्रपीडनात्।

मज्जवाहीनि दुष्यन्ति विरुद्धानां च सेवनात्। (च. वि. 5/18)

मज्जावहस्रोतो दुष्टिलक्षणानि

रुक् पर्वणां भ्रमो मूर्च्छा दर्शनं तमसस्तथा।

अरुषां स्थूलमूलानां पर्वजानां च दर्शनम्।

मज्जाप्रदोषात्।– (च. सू. 28/17)

चिकित्सा

मज्जशुक्रसमुत्थानामौषधं स्वादुतिक्तकम्।

अन्नं व्यवायव्यायामौ शुद्धि: काले च मात्रया। (च. सू. 28/28)

शुक्रवह स्रोतस्

शुक्रवहानां स्रोतसां वृषणौ मूलं शेफश्च। (च. वि. 5/8)

शुक्रवहे द्वे, तयोर्मूलं स्तनौ वृक्षणौ च। (सु. शा. 9/12)

शुक्रवहस्रोतो दुष्टिकारणानि

अकालयोनिगमनान्निनिग्रहातिमैथुनात्।

शुक्रवाहीनि दुष्यन्ति शस्त्रक्षाराग्निभिस्तथा। (च. वि. 5/19)

शुक्रवहस्रोतो दुष्टिलक्षणानि

शुक्रस्य दोषात् क्लैब्यमहर्षणम्।

रोगी वा क्लीबमल्पायुर्विरूपं वा प्रजायते।

न चास्य जायते गर्भ: पतित प्रस्रवत्यपि।

शुक्रं हि दुष्टं सापत्यं सदारं बाधते नरम्।। (च. सू. 28/18, 19)

विद्धलक्षणानि

तत्र विद्धस्य क्लीबता चिरात्प्रसेको रक्तशुक्रता च। (सु. शा. 9/12)

चिकित्सा

मज्जशुक्रसमुत्थानातमौषधं स्वादुतिक्तकम्।

अन्नं व्यवासव्यायामौ शुद्धि: काले च मात्रया।   (च. सू. 28/28)

मूत्रवहस्रोतस्

मूत्रवहे द्वे, तयोर्मूलं बस्तिर्मेढ्रं च।   (सु. शा. 9/12)

मूत्रहानां स्रोतसां बस्तिर्मूलं वङ्क्षणौ च।   (च. वि. 5/8)

मूत्रवहस्रोतो दुष्टिकारणानि

मूत्रितोदकभक्ष्यस्त्रीसेवनान्मूनिग्रहात्।

मूत्रवाहिनी दुष्यन्ति क्षीणस्याभिक्षतस्य च।   (च. वि. 5/20)

मूत्रवहस्रोतो दुष्टिलक्षणानि

अतिसृष्टमतिबद्धं कुपितमल्पाल्पमभीक्ष्णं वा बहलं सशब्दशूलमूच्छ्वसन्तं दृष्ट्वा

प्राणवहान्यस्य मूत्रवहान्यस्य स्रोतांसि प्रदुष्टानीति विद्यात्।   (च. वि. 5/8)

विद्धलक्षणानि

तत्र विद्धस्यानद्धबस्तिता मूत्रनिरोध: स्तब्धमेढ्रता च।   (सू. शा. 9/12)

चिकित्सा

मूत्रविट्स्वेदवाहानां चिकित्सा मौत्रकृच्छ्रकी।

तथाऽतिसारिकी कार्या तथा ज्वरचिकित्सिकी।।   (च. वि. 5/28)

पुरीषवहस्रोतस्

पुरीषवहानां स्रोतसा पक्वाशयो मूलं स्थुलगुदं च।   (च. वि. 5/8)

पुरीषवहे द्वे, तयोर्मूलं पक्वाशयो गुदं च।   (सू. शा. 9/12)

पुरीषवहस्रोतो दुष्टिलकारणानि

सन्धारणादत्यशनादजीर्णाध्यशनात् तथा।

वर्चोवाहिनि दुष्यन्ति दुर्बलाग्ने: कृशस्य च।।   (च. वि. 5/21)

पुरीषवहस्रोतोह दुष्टिलक्षणानि

कृच्छ्रेणाल्पाल्पं सशब्दशूलमतिद्रवमतिग्रथितमतिबहु चोपविशन्तं दृष्ट्वा

पुरीषवहान्यस्य स्रोतांसि प्रदुष्टानीति विद्यात्।   (च. वि. 5/8)

विद्धलक्षणानि

तत्र विद्धस्यानहो दुर्गन्धता ग्रथितान्नता च।   (सु. शा. 9/12)

चिकित्सा

नवेगान्धारणेऽध्याये चिकित्सासङ्ग्रह: कृत:।

मलजानां विकाराणां सिद्धिश्चोक्ता क्वचित् त्क्वचित्।।   (च. सू. 28/30)

स्वेदवह स्रोतस्

स्वेदवहानां स्रोतसा मेदो मूलं लोमकूपाश्च।   (च. वि. 5/8)

स्वेदवहस्रोता दुष्टिकारणानि

व्यायामादतिसन्तापाच्छीतोष्णाक्रमसेवनात्।

स्वेदवाहीनि दुष्यन्ति क्रोधशोकभयैस्तथा।।   (च. वि. 5/22)

स्वेदवहस्रोतो दुष्टिलक्षणानि

अस्वेदनमतिस्वेदं पारुष्यमतिश्लक्षणतामङ्गस्य परिदाहं लोमहर्ष च दृष्ट्वा
स्वेदवहान्यस्य स्रोतांसि प्रदुष्टानीति विद्यात्।   (च. वि. 5/8)

चिकित्सा

मूत्रविट्स्वेदवहानां चिकित्सा मौत्रकृच्छ्रिकी।

तथाऽतिसारिकी कार्या तथा ज्वरचिकित्सकी।।   (च. वि. 9/28)

आर्तववहस्रोतस्

आर्तववहे द्वे, तयोर्मूलं गर्भाशय-आर्तववाहिन्यश्च।

धमन्य:।   (सु. शा. 9/12)

विद्धलक्षणानि

तत्र विद्धायां वन्ध्यात्वं मैथुनासहिष्णुत्वमार्त्तवनाशश्च।   (सु. शा. 9/12)

चिकित्सा

कायचिकित्सायां तु स्रोतोरोध एव प्राधान्येन रोगाणां कारणम्। तत्र स्रोतोमुखविशोधनात्
दोषा: कोष्ठं यान्ति अनन्तरं विनिहरेत्। एषा शोधनचिकित्सा।

(च. सू. 28/5; आ. श. भा. 2; पृ. 1683)

6
DIGESTIVE AND TISSUE ENZYMES
(AGNI)

The energy or the heat element exists in the body in the form of *Pitta*, i.e. various enzymes. Health, vigour, strength and life itself depends on the digestive and tissue enzymes. Abnormal activity of these enzymes leads to disease while cessation of activity leads to death. A person with good digestive power, i.e. *sama-agni* will have good appetite, can digest even heavy food items like *shrikand*, chicken, payasam, etc. without having any symptoms of indigestion. After digestion of food, it is responsible for formation of various constituents of the body namely various tissue enzymes as well as *doshas*.

CLASSIFICATION OF ENZYMES, I.E. AGNI

(1) *Jatharagni* or *Pachakagni*, which is respresented by the digestive enzymes.

(2) *Dhatvagni*, i.e. tissue enzymes.

(3) *Bhutagni*, i.e. elemental enzymes responsible for digestion of five basic elements, viz. earth by *bhoumagni*, water by *apyagni*, energy by *agneyagni*, air by *vayavyagni* and Space by *nabhasagni*. By digestion of energy element, one means transfer of energy into utilisable form. The food is composed of all the five basic elements and individual elements in the food are digested by their corresponding *bhutagni*, i.e. elemental enzymes.

CAUSES OF AFFECTION OF DIGESTIVE AND TISSUE ENZYMES

(1) Dietetic causes, i.e. eating in excess, fasting, incom-

patible diet, diet to which one is not used to heavy, cold, dry or unclean diet, unbalanced diet, etc.

(2) Iatrogenic causes, i.e. administration of emetices, purgatives or any other medicine in an inappropriate manner.

(3) During and following any disease.

(4) Environmental factors like abnormal seasons, hot and moist climate.

(5) Suppression of natural urges.

(6) Abnormal *doshas*.

(7) Diseases of digestive tract.

(8) Constitutional causes.

The digestive power is classified as follows :

(1) *Vishama* : Irregular due to *Vata* predominance.

(2) *Tikshna* : Sharp due to *Pitta* predominance.

(3) *Manda* : Weak due to *Kapha* predominance.

(4) *Sama* : Balanced due fo balanced state of *Vata*, *Pitta* and *Kapha*.

Vishamagni : It results from diet and activities increasing *Vata dosha*, which vitiates the digestive enzymes and gives rise to *Vataja* disorders. A person with *vishama* or irregular digestive power has variable digestive power. Sometimes, the digestion is good and at other times he suffers from distension, constipation, diarrhoea, heaviness of abdomen, borborygmi, colicky pain, tenesmus, etc. due to indigestion. Such a person is prone to develop *Vata* disorders. He should take predominantly unctuous food with sour and salty taste. He should take *tila* oil enema intermittently.

Tikshnagni : It results from diet and activities increasing *Pitta dosha* which vitiates the digestive enzymes and gives rise to *Pittaja* disorders. People with sharp digestive power digest their food very quickly. It is termed as *atyaagni,* when the digestive power is abnormally increased. Such a person digests even large quantities of food and later emaciates because of increased quantity of tissue enzymes and raised metabolic rate. Such an individual is prone to *Pitta* disorders like hyperacidity, diarrhoea, etc. He should take predominantly sweet, unctuous and cold food. He should take purgatives intermittently.

Mandagni : It results from diet and activities increasing *Kapha dosha* and gives rise to *Kapha* disorders. The *Kapha dosha* vitiates the digestive enzymes. Persons with weak digestive power take a long time to digest even a small quantity of food. They commonly suffer from heaviness, cough, breathlessness, drooling of saliva, nausea and a state of exhaustion after eating food. Such persons are prone to *Kapha* disorders. They should take food with predominantly bitter, pungent or astringent taste. They should take emetics intermittently.

Samagni : A person with ideal or balanced digestive power digests food easily and does not suffer from digestive disorders even with food irregularities. He can tolerate hunger as well as excessive food intake well. Even then one should try to preserve the digestive power of such a person. *Prana vayu* helps ingestion of food, *Samana vayu* controls peristaltic activity and absorption of food, and *apana vayu* controls defaecation and expulsion of gases.

All the diseases arise as a result of less, excessive or abnormal digestive or tissue enzymes. Weak digestive power lowers the body resistance and acts as a predisposing factor to all the diseases. Even if the germs of various diseases enter the body, viz. food and water contaminated by flies, faeces etc. the germs are killed by the acid in the stomach and the digestive juices in the gastro-instestinal tract. In case they enter and circulate in the body, they are inactivated by the active tissue enzymes. Hence, a person with weak digestive power and inadequate issue enzymes is predisposed to various diseases.

अग्नि:

मरिचिरुवाच– अग्निरेव शरीरे पित्तान्तर्गत: कुपिताकुपित: शुभाशुभानि करोति।
तद्यथा–पक्तिमपक्तिं दर्शनमदर्शनं मात्रत्वमूष्मण: प्रकृतिविकृवर्णौशौर्यं भयं क्रोधं
हर्षं मोहं प्रसादमित्येवमादीनि चापराणि द्वन्द्वानिति।।   (च. सू. 12/11)

न खलुपित्तव्यतिरेकादन्योऽग्निरूपलभ्यते।।   (सु. सू. 21/9)

आयुर्वर्णोबलं स्वास्थ्यमुत्साहोपचयौ प्रभा। ओजस्तेजोऽग्नय: प्राणाश्चोक्ता
देहाग्निहेतुका:।।

शान्तेऽग्नौ म्रियते, युक्ते चिरंवत्यनामय:। रोगी स्याद्विकृते, मूलमग्नितस्मा-
न्निरुच्यते।।   (च. चि. 15/4)

अनस्य पक्ता पित्तं तु पाचकाख्यं पुरेरितम्। दोषधातुमलादिनामूष्मेत्यात्रेयशासनम्।।
          (अ. हृ. शा. 3)

पाचकपित्तम्

......................तत्र पक्कामाशयमध्यगम्। पञ्चभूतात्मकत्वेऽपि
यत्तैजसगुणोदयात्।।

त्यक्तद्रवत्त्वं पाकादिकर्मणाऽनलशब्दितम्। पचत्यन्नं विभजते सारकिट्टौ पृथक् तथा।।

तत्रस्थमेव पित्तानां शेषाणामष्यनुग्रहम्। करोति बलदानेन पाचकं नाम तत् स्मृतम्।।
          (अ. हृ. सू. 12/10–12)

अग्निविचार:

स्वस्थानस्थस्य कायोग्नेरंशा धातुषु संश्रिता:। तेषां सादातिदीप्तिभ्यां धातुवृद्धि-
क्षयोद्भव:।।   (अ. हृ. सू. 11/34)

भौमाप्याग्नेयवायव्या: पञ्चोष्माण: सनाभसा:। पञ्चाहारगुणान्स्वान्स्वान्पार्थिवा-
दिन्पचन्तिहि।।

यथास्वं स्वं च पुष्णन्ति देहे द्रव्यगुणा: पृथक्। पार्थिवा: पार्थिवानेव शेषा: शेषांश्च
कृत्स्नशा:।।   (च. चि. 15/13–14)

रोगा: सर्वेऽपि मन्देऽग्नौ सुतरामुदराणि च।।   (अ. हृ. नि. 12/1)

7

DIETETIC FACTORS
(AHARAJA KARANANI)

Diet is important for maintenance of health. However, if one does not use his discretion regarding selection of his food in relation to place, time, constitution, etc. as given below, the same diet can give rise to disease by vitiating the *doshas* :

(1) *Diet and Place* : Eating hot and pungent food in continental climate *(Jangala desh)* or eating fatty and cold food items in maritime climate would increase *Pitta* and *Kapha doshas* respectively.

(2) *Diet and Season* : Eating hot and pungent food in summer or cold food in winter would increase *Pitta* and *Kapha doshas* respectively.

(3) *Quantity and Quality* : Eating heavy food items in excess or too less quantity of food of light items would increase *Kapha* and *Vata doshas* respectively.

(4) Eating food to which one is not habituated would also cause sudden imbalance of *doshas*.

(5) *Constitution and Diet* : If a person with *Vata* constitution eats dry food, person with *Pitta* constitution eats hot and pungent food and person with *Kapha* constitution eats fatty and sweet food in excess, it would result in increase of the same *dosha* in his body.

(6) *Diet and Digestive Power* : If a person with weak digestive power eats heavy food items, it leads to formation of *ama*.

(7) *Diet and Srotorodha* : Diet which increase *doshas* and simultaneously damage tissues leads to obstruction of the body channels.

(8) *Dietetic Incompatibilities* : Eating combination of milk and fish will result in increased amount of *doshas* in the body.

(9) *Eating Raw Food Items in Excess* : Raw ood items which are difficult to digest such as green leafy vegetables would increase *Vata dosha* in the body.

(10) *Psychological Incompatibility* : One should not eat food items which one does not like.

(11) One should not eat fermented and putrefied food or food which is not freshly prepared.

(12) *Time* : Eating food at irregular hours or eating food when not hungry makes a person prone to disease.

Our ancient masters have studied elaborately the qualities of each and every food preparation and their effect on the tissues of healthy as well as diseased individuals of various constitutions. Hence, we find references of dietary factors as aetiological factors which trigger off subdue as well as aggravate many disease processes. Hence, in almost all diseases Ayurveda advises the avoidance of certain food items, which have a tendency to aggravate the disease and consumption of certain food items that have a beneficial effect on the recovery from the disease.

आहारजकारणानि

आहारजवातप्रकोपहेतवः

कटुतिक्तकषायरुक्षलघुशीतवीर्य शुष्कशाक वल्लूरवर कोद्दालक कोरदूषश्यामाक नीवारमुद्गमसूराढकीहरेणुकलायनिष्पावानशनाध्यशनात् वायुः प्रकोपमापद्यते ।।

(सु. सू. 21/19)

तिक्तोष्णकषायरस सेवनैः .... समीरण: कुप्यति ।

(अ. सं. नि. 1)

पित्तप्रकोप हेतवः (आहारज)

उष्णाम्ललवण क्षारकटुकाजीर्ण भोजनेभ्योऽतिसेवितेभ्यः तीक्ष्णातपाग्निसन्तापश्रम-क्रोधविषमाहारेभ्यः पित्तं प्रकोपमापद्यते ।। (च. नि. 1/22)

कट्वम्ललवणतीक्ष्णोष्णलघुविदाहितिलतैलपिण्याककुलत्थ सर्षपातसीहरीतकीशाक गोधामत्स्याजाविकमांसदधितक्रकूर्चिकामस्तुसौवीरक सुराविकाराम्ल कट्वरभृतिभिः पित्तं प्रकोपमापद्यते ।। (सु. सू. 21/20)

श्लेष्मप्रकोपहेतव: (आहारज)

मधुराम्ललवणशीत, स्निग्धगुरुपिच्छिल, अभिष्यन्दि हायनकथवक नैषधेत्कट
माषमहामाष गोधूम तिल, पिष्ट, विकृति दधि दुग्ध कृशरा पायस इक्षु विकारानू-
पौदकमांसवसा बिसमृणालकसेरुक शृङ्गाटक मधुवल्लीफल समशनाध्यशन-
प्रभृतिभि: श्लेष्माप्रकोपमापद्यते ।।   (सु. सू. 23/22)

स्वाद्वम्ललवणस्निग्धगुर्वभिष्यन्दशीतलै:।   (अ. हृ. नि. 1/17)

आहार:

यच्चापि देशकालाग्निमात्रासात्म्यानिलादिभि:। संस्कारतो वीर्यतश्च कोष्ठा-
वस्थाक्रमैरपि ।।

परिहारोपचाराभ्यां पाकात् संयोगतोऽपि च। विरुद्धं तच्च न हितं हृत्सम्पद्विधिभिश्च
यत्।।

विरुद्धं देशतस्तावद् रुक्षतीक्ष्णादि धन्वनि। आनूपे स्निग्धशीतादि भेषजं यन्निषेध्यते।।

कालतोऽपि विरुद्धं यच्छीतरुक्षादि सेवनम्। शीते काले, तथोष्णे च कटुकोष्णा-
दिसेवनम्।।

विरुद्धमनले तद्वन्नपानं चतुर्विधे। मधुसर्पि: समघृतं मात्रया तद्विरुध्यते।।

कटुकोष्णादिसात्म्यस्य स्वादुशीतादिसेवनम्। यत्तत्सात्म्यविरुद्धं तु विरुद्ध
त्वनिलादिभि:।।

या समानगुणाभ्यासविरुद्धानौषधक्रिया। संस्कारतो विरुद्धं तद् तद्भोज्यं विषवद्भवेत्।।

ऐरण्डसीसकासक्तं शिखिमांसं तथैव हि। विरुद्धं वीर्यतो ज्ञेयं वीर्य: शीतलात्मकम्।।

तत् संयोज्योष्णवीर्येण द्रव्येण सह सेव्यते। क्रूरकोष्ठस्य चात्यल्पं मन्दवीर्यमभेदनम्।।

मृदुकोष्ठस्य गुरुच भेदनीयं तथा बहु। एतत्कोष्ठविरुद्धं तु, विरुद्धं स्यादवस्थया।।

श्रमव्यवायव्यायामसक्तस्यानिलकोपनम्। निद्रालसस्यालसस्य भोजनं श्लेष्मकोपनम्।।

यच्चानुत्सृज्य विण्मूत्रं भुंक्ते यश्चाबुभुक्षित:। तच्च क्रमविरुद्ध स्याद्यच्या-
तिक्षुद्रशानुग:।।

परिहारविरुद्धं तु वराहादीनिषेव्य यत्। सेवेतोष्णं, घृतादीश्चं पीत्वा शीतं निषेवते।।

विरुद्धं पाकतश्चापि दुष्टदुर्द्रारुसाधितम्। अपक्वतण्डुलाव्यर्थपक्वदग्धं च यद् भवेत्।।

संयोगतो विरुद्धं तद्यथाऽम्लं पयसा सह। अमनोरुचितं यच्च हृद् विरुद्धं तदुच्यते।।

सम्पद्विरुद्धं तद्विद्याादसञ्जातरसं तु यत्। अतिक्रान्तरसं वाऽपि विपन्नरसमेव वा।।

ज्ञेयं विधिविरुद्धं तु भुज्यते निभृते न यत्। तदेवं विधमन्नं स्याद् विरुद्धमुपयोजितम्।।

सात्म्यतोऽल्पतया वाऽपि दीप्ताग्नेस्तरुणस्य च। स्निग्धव्यायामबलिनो विरुद्धं वितथं
भवेत्।।   (च. सू. अ. 26)

8
TOXINS
(AMA)

During digestion the food is broken down into smaller and smaller particles till they are broken down ultimately into fine particles, which can be easily absorbed and assimilated. Incompletely digested food products which cannot be absorbed, remain in the gastro-intestinal tract and are passed in the stools or vomited. The partially digested food which can be absorbed, but cannot be assimilated by tissues is termed as *ama*.

When the amount of food taken is beyond one's digestive capacity, it leads to formation of *ama*. Thus, a person with good digestive power will hardly ever form *ama*. On the other hand, a person with weak digestive power quickly forms *ama*, even if he takes limited or moderate amount of food stuff. *Ama* is also formed when *doshas* affect each other. In *dvandvaja* and *tridoshaja* diseases, more than one *doshas* are increased in the body and affect the tissue. In these conditions, *doshas* do not affect each other. When the increased *doshas* attack each other i.e. combine chemically with each other, the result is the formation of *ama,* i.e. a toxic chemical compound. *Ama* formed in this manner is highly toxic to the tissues and is encountered in states of toxemia and other fulminating diseases affecting the entire body.

Table showing formation of *Ama* from incomplete digestion of food.

Diet	Digestive–Power	Tissue–enzymes	Remarks
• +	+	+	Formation of tissues, normal *doshas* and wast products in appropriate amounts

Diet	Digestive–Power	Tissue–enzymes	Remarks
• Slightly more +	+	+	Fat, *doshas* and waste products in increased amount
• ++	+	+	*Ama* formation in gastro-intestinal tract
• +	+	—	*Ama* formation in tissues
• +	–	+	*Ama* formation in gastro-intestinal tract
• ++	++	+	*Ama* formation in tissues
• +++	+	+	*Ama* + undigested food in gastro-intestinal tract

Ama is one of the important cause of majority of diseases. The first variety of *ama* resulting from incomplete digestion of food accumulate, slowly in genetically weak organs or organs weakened by obstruction to its blood vessels or its ducts and gives rise to sub-acute or chronic diseases. The *ama* can affect *doshas*, tissues or waste products.

When *ama* afflicts various *doshas*, they are termed as *sama doshas*. Thus, one gets *sama Vata, sama Pitta* and *sama Kapha*. The stage of disease where *ama doshas* dominate is termed as *sama* stage of disease. When these *ama doshas* are digested either by tissue enzymes or by enzymes in the digestive tract, one gets rid of *ama doshas* and this is termed as *nirama* stage of the disease.

CHARACTERS OF TOXINS (AMA)

It is heavy, unctuous, viscid, foul smelling and toxic fluid. It contain fine thread like material. It can have many colours and is the root cause of al illnesses.

General symptoms due to *ama doshas* are as follows :

Obstruction to passages, improper functioning of heart, weakness, heaviness obstruction to the free movement and functioning of *Vata*; laziness, drowsiness indigestion, heaviness in stomach, expectoration, retention of urine and stools anorexia and exhaustion. The pulse is heavy, slow and strong. Urine is slimy, foul smelling, of varying colours and has high specific gravity. Stools may, have shades of various colours. It is foul smelling and sinks in water. Tongue is slimy and heavily coated, the coating being difficult to remove by cleaning the tongue.

One may get *ama* stage in relation to *dosha,* i.e. *Vata, Pitta, Kapha* and *dhatus,* i.e. body fluids, blood, etc. and *malas,* i.e. waste products.

Symptoms of Sama Vata and Nirama Vata : Pain of various types, gaseous destension, weak digestive power, constipation oedema, drowsiness or disturbed functions of *Vata* are the symptoms of *sama Vata.* The symptoms of *Sama Vata* are increased by administration of oils and ghee. Sense of clarity and dryness, free passage of wind and stools, dimunition in the severity of pain and its relief by medicated oil and ghee are the manifestations of *nirama Vata.*

Symptoms of Sama and Nirama Pitta : *Sama Pitta* is foul smelling, greenish-black, sour, heavy and steady. It is usually secreted in profuse amount and gives rise to burning in throat and cardiac region.

Nirama Pitta is reddish-yellow, hot, pungent, mobile and does not have any smell. It imparts digestive power, taste and strength.

Symptoms of Sama and Nirama Kapha : *Sama Kapha* is heavy, viscid, thick, foul smelling, turbid, dirty and thready. It destroys appetite and impairs easy belching.

Nirama Kapha becomes clear, foamy, white, sweet and does not have foul smell. It imparts a clean sensation to the mouth and throat.

TREATMENT OF AMA DOSHAS

Fasting is the best method of treatment of *ama* stage of any disease. One should undertake the fast till *ama* is digested, i.e. the symptoms of *ama* or indigestion disappear and one feels light. The administration of medicine is contraindicated in this stage, as the medicine itself may not, be digested and may exert local irritant action or exhibit abnormal toxic symptoms. At the most, one may administer medicines, which will act as digestives or stimulate secretion of digestive juice. In case the patient has nausea and retching, one should administer an emetic. Purgatives are usually contraindicated as the toxins of *ama* driven into the intestine then can be easily absorbed leading to toxaemia.

If *ama dosha* is naturally getting out of the body, e.g. in *ama* stage of vomiting and diarrhoea, one should not interfere with it by administering anti-emetic or astringent medicines. This may lead to retention of toxins and a state of toxaemia. Fasting is also indicated, when *ama doshas* have accumulated in the tissues or has spread all over the body as in states of toxaemia. One should get rid of *ama* by stimulating the tissue enzymes, which would digest *ama* locally. Later, one should bring the digested *doshas* to the gastro-intestinal tract by administration of medicated oils and ghee and induction of sweating. Finally, these *doshas* in the gastro-intestinal tract should be removed from the body by administration of emetics, purgatives or enema.

आम:

सामावस्था

उष्मणोऽल्पबलत्वेन धातुमाद्यमपाचितम्।

दुष्टमामाशयगतं रसमामं प्रचक्षते।।

आमेन तेन सम्पृक्ता दोषा दूष्याश्च दूषिता:।

सामा इत्युपदिश्यन्ते ये च रोगास्तदुद्भवा:।।

अन्ये दोषेभ्य एवाति दुष्टेभ्योऽन्योन्यमूर्च्छनात्।

कोद्रवेभ्यो विषस्येव वदन्त्यामस्य सम्भवम्।　　　（अ. ह. सू. 13/25-27)

स:- अन्ये-अपरे आचार्या:, दोषेभ्यएव-वातादिभ्यो, अतिदुष्टेभ्योऽन्योन्यमूर्च्छनात्-

परस्परमिश्रीभावात्, आमस्य संभवं कथयन्ति। केभ्य: कस्येव? यथा कोद्रवेभ्यो विषस्य सम्भवं कथन्ति। (तथा दोषभ्य आमस्य संभवम्।)

आ. र: -मतान्तरेणामलक्षणमाह-अन्य इति अन्योन्यमूच्छर्नात्-परस्पर- मेकलोलीभावात्।

(अ. हृ. सू. 13/26; निदानपञ्चक सम्प्राप्तिविज्ञान पृ. 128)

सामनिराम सामान्य लक्षणानि

स्रोतोरो द्घबलभ्रंशगौरवानिलमूढता:।
आलस्यपक्तिनिष्ठीवमलसंगारुचिक्लमा:।
लिङ्गं मलानां सामानां निरामाणां विपर्यय:।

सामनिरामवायो: लक्षणानि

विरचेदयुगपच्चापिगृह्णाति कुपितोभृशम्।
स्नेहाद्यैर्वृद्धि माप्नोति सूर्य-मेघोदये निशि।।
वायु: सामो विबन्धाग्निसादस्तन्द्रान्त्रकूजनै:।
वेदनाशोथनिस्तोदै: क्रमशोऽङ्गानि पीडयेत्।।
निरामो विशदो रुक्षो निर्विबन्धोऽल्पवेदन:।
विपरीतगुणै: शांति स्निग्धैर्यात्ति विशेषत:।।

सामनिरामपित्तयो: लक्षणानि

दुर्गन्ध हरितं श्यावं पित्तमम्लं स्थिरं गुरु।
आम्लिकाकण्ठ हृद्दाहकरं सामं विनिर्दिशेत्।
आताम्रं पीतमत्युष्णं रसे कटुकमस्थिरम्।
पक्वं विगन्धं विज्ञेयं रुचिपक्तृबलप्रदम्।।

सामनिरामकफयो: लक्षणानि

अविलस्तन्तुलस्त्यान: कण्ठेदेशेऽवतिष्ठते।
सामो बलासो दुर्गन्ध: क्षुदुद्गारविघातकृत्।।
फेनवान्पिण्डित: पाण्डुर्नि:सारोऽगन्ध एव च।
पक्व: स एव विज्ञेयश्छेदवान्वक्त्रशुद्धिकृत्।।

(मा. नि. 5, टीका. पृ. 10-11; नि. पं. सं. वि. पृ. 126, 127)

लङ्घनचिकित्सा

आमाशयस्थो हत्वाऽग्निं सामो मार्गान् पिधाय यत्।
विदधाति ज्वरं दोषस्तस्मात्कुर्वीत लङ्घनम्।।
विदधाति ज्वरादौ वा बलं यत्नेन पालयन्।
बलाधिष्ठानमारोग्यमरोग्यार्थ: क्रियामक:।।   (अ. ह. चि.1/1-2)
प्रवृत्तान् प्रागतो दोषानुपेक्षेत हिताशिन:।।
विबद्धान् पावनैस्तैस्तै: पाचयेन्निहरेत वा।।   (अ. ह. सू. 13/32)
उत्क्लिष्ट्यानध ऊर्ध्व वा न चामान् वहत: स्वयम्।।
धारयेदौषधे: दोषान् विधृतास्ते हि रोगदा:।   (अ. ह. सू. 13/31)

सामदोषचिकित्सा

सर्वदेहप्रविसृतान् सामान् दोषान् निहरेत्।
लीनान् धातुष्वनुत्क्लिष्ट्यान् फलादामाद्रसानिव।।
आश्रयस्य हि नाशाय ते स्युर्दुर्निर्हरत्वत:।
पाचनैर्दीपनै: स्नेहैस्तान् स्वेदैश्च परिष्कृतान्।।
शोधयेच्छाधनै: काले यथासन्नं यथाबलम्।
हन्त्याशु युक्तं वक्त्रेण द्रव्यमामाशयान्मलान्।।
घ्राणेन चोर्ध्वजत्रूत्थान् पक्वाधनाद गुदेन च।   (अ. ह. सू. 13/28-30)

9

INFECTIOUS DISEASES
AND PARASITIC INFESTATIONS
(KRIMIROGA)

Germs and parasites are of two types, i.e. external and internal.

External Germs and Parasites, i.e. Bahyakrimi : Unclean habits promote the growth of these germs and parasites. They are minute, invisible or microscopic in size. They are white or black in colour. *Yuka,* i.e. lice and *pipilika,* i.e. ant-like parasites of scabies and other microscopic *krimis* affect hair and skin.

Internal Germs and Parasities, i.e. Abhyantara : They are divided into : (i) *Raktaja krimi,* i.e. germs and parasite in blood, (ii) *Shleshmaja krimi,* i.e. germs and parasites in the region where *Kapha* dominates and (iii) *Purishaja krimi,* i.e. germs and parasites in faeces.

(i) *Raktaja Krimi* : These germs and parasites are termed as : — (a) *Keshada,* i.e. those eating hair, (b) *Lomada,* i.e. thriving on body hair, (c) *Nakhada,* i.e. thriving on nails (d) *Dantada,* i.e. thriving on teeth and which to leads to caries of teeth, (e) *Kikkisa,* (f) *Kushtaja,* (g) *Praisarpa,* (h) *Lomadvipa,* (i) *Sourasa,* (j) *Udumbara,* and (k) *Jantumatru,* causing various sking diseases. These parasites are very minute and round in shape. They are present in the blood. The factors leading to skin diseases promote the growth of these parasites.

(ii) *Shleshmaja or Kaphaja Krimi* : These parasites thrive on *Kapha.* The growth of these parasites is promoted by taking in excess milk, jaggery *tila,* pulses, *udid,* leafy vegetables, meat of aquatic animals, sweets, curds, oil, starchy food, sunflower oil, indigested, stale, rotten and dirty food and incompatible diet. These parasites initially arise in stomach and later can affect the areas where *Kapha* dominates. They are white or red in colour, flat, round or elongated in shape and minute or microscopic in size. Their names are *antrada,* i.e. thriving on small intestine, *udarad,* i.e. thriving in abdomen, *hridayachara,* i.e. thriving on heart, *darbhapushpi,* i.e. having a big anus, *praluna,* i.e. rounded *chipita,* flat *pipilaka,* i.e. resembling an ant and *daruna,* i.e. those leading to severe sickness. These germs and parasites affect brain, eyes, palate and ears and give rise to headache, fever, anorexia, indigestion, fainting, unconsciousness, yawning, sneezing, colds, vomiting, distension, loss of weight and stiffness of the body.

Treatment : The treatment consists of (a) Administration of medicines, which will act on the causative germs or parasites. The diet and medicines should be dominant in bitter, pungent, astringent and hot qualities. (b) *Apakarshana,* i.e. expulsion of worms by administration of milk, curds, *tila,* fish, meat of aquatic animals, starchy food, etc. in the dinner. These dietetic factors attract the germs and parasites and thus, the hold of the worms on the intestine is loosened. This is followed by administration of emetics, purgatives and enema next morning. Local cleansing medications should be administered to get rid off local germs and parasites, e.g. cleansing nasal medication and cleansing eye-wash. (c) Prevention of recurrence by avoiding the aetiological factors.

Medical Treatment : (a) Fresh juice or paste of *palashabija* should be taken with rice-water. (b) Fresh juice of leaves of *paribhadraka,* i.e. *parvatanimba* should be taken with honey. (c) Fresh juice of *pattura* or *surasadi* group of medicines should be taken with honey. (d) *Vidanga* should be given by mouth.

Tilvaka, karanja, mustard, *koshataki, shyama, chavya, chitraka, bhringaraja, kadamba, surasa, pudina, apamarga, kutaja, bakula, svarnakshiri, mushkaparni, pippali, kushtha, kutaki,* ginger, *daruharidra, kulattha kshara* and *yavakshara* also act on germs and parasites. For the treatment of *raktaja krimi,* i.e. germs and parasites in the blood, you may refer to the chapter on treatment of skin diseases in the Ayurvedic texts.

(iii) *Parasites in Faces, i.e. Purishaja Krimi* : The causative factors are the same as the *Kaphaja* parasites. These germs and parasites are present in small and large intestines, and vary in size from minute to macroscopic. They may be flat, round or cylindrical. The colour may black, blue, green or yellow. Their names are *Gandupada,* i.e. round worms, *ajava,* i.e. worms with slow movement, *vijava,* i.e. with fast movement, *kipya, chipya, churu, dvimukha, kakeruka, makeruka, lehika,* i.e. those which lick the intestines, *shulaka,* i.e. worms giving rise to pain and *sousurada.* These parasites and germs give rise to diarrhoea, emaciation, goose-skin, itching of the anus, pain in the abdomen, fever, anaemia, giddiness, anorexia, heart diseases and weakness.

कृमिरोगा:

निदान-(पुरीषजानां कृमीणां)

अजीर्णाध्यशनासात्म्यविरुद्धमलिनाशनै:।
अव्यायामदिवास्वप्नगुर्वतिस्निग्धशीतलै:॥
माषपिष्टान्नविदलबिसशालूकसेरुकै:।
पर्णशाकसुराशुक्तदधिक्षीरगुडेधुभि:॥
पललानूपपिशितपिण्याकपृथुकादिभि:।
स्वाद्म्लद्रवपानैश्च श्लेष्मा पित्तञ्च कुप्यति॥
कृमीन् बहुविधाकारान् करोति विविधाश्रयान्।   (सु. उ. 54/3-5)

संख्या

पुरीषजा:, श्लेष्मजा:, शोणितजा:, मलजाश्चेति॥
विंशते: कृमिजातीनां त्रिविध: सम्भव: स्मृत:।   (च. वि. 7/9)
पुरीषकुरक्तानि तासां वक्ष्यामि विस्तरम्।   (सु. उ. 54/7)
विंशतिकृमिजातय इति-यूका: पिपीलिकाश्चेति द्विविधाबहिर्मलजा:, केशादा, लोमादा

सोमद्वीपा: सौरसा औदुम्बरजन्तुमातरश्चेतिषट्शोणितजा:, अन्त्रादाउदरवावेष्टा
हृदयादाश्रुखो दर्भपुष्पा: सौगन्धिकामहा गुदाश्चेतिसप्त कफजा, कसेरुकामकेरु-
कालेलिहा: सशूलका: सौसुरादाश्चेति पञ्च पुरीषजा:।।   (च. वि. 8/9)

अजवा विजवा: किप्याश्चिप्पा गण्डूपदास्तथा।

चूर्वो द्विमुखाश्चैव ज्ञेया: सप्त पुरीषजा:।।   (सु. उ. 54/8)

तत्रमलो बाह्यश्चाभ्यान्तरश्च तत्र बाह्यमलजातान् मलजान् सङ्क्ष्महे। तेषां
समुत्थानं-मृजावर्जनं-स्थानं; केशश्मश्रुलोमपक्ष्मवासांसि; संस्थानम्-अणवस्ति-
लाकृतयो बहुपादाश्च, वर्ण:-कृष्ण: शुक्लश्च।।   (च. वि. 7)

स्थानम्

आमपक्वाशये तेषां कफविड्जन्मतां पुन:।

धमन्यांरक्तजानां च प्रसव: प्रायश: स्मृत:।।   (सु. उ. 54/6)

तेषां स्थानं पक्वाशय:, ते प्रवर्धमाना: तु अधोविसर्पन्ति, यस्य पुनरामाशयाभिमुखा:।

लक्षणम्

श्वेता: सूक्ष्मास्तुदन्त्येते गुदं प्रतिसरन्ति च।

तेषामेवापरे पुच्छै: पृथवश्च भवन्ति हि।।

शूलाग्निमान्द्यपाण्डुत्वविष्टम्भबलसङ्क्षया:।

प्रसेकारुचिहृद्रोगविड्भेदास्तु पुरीषजै:।।   (सु. उ. 54/9-10)

यस्य पुनरामाशयाभिमुखा: स्युर्मदन्तरं तदन्तरं तस्योद्गारनि:श्वासा: पुरीषगन्धिन:
स्यु:।   (च. वि. 7)

संस्थानवर्णविशेषास्तु-सूक्ष्मवृत्तपरीणाहा:, श्वेता दीर्घाऊर्णा शुसङ्काशा: केचित्, केचित्
पुन: स्थूलवृत्तपरीणाहा:; श्यावनीलहरीतपीता:।।   (च. वि. 7/13)

प्रभाव:

पुरीषभेद:, काश्र्यं, पारुष्यं, लोमहर्षाभिनिर्वर्तनं च, त एव चास्य गुदुमुखं
परितुदन्त:, कण्डुं चोपजनयन्तो गुदमुखं पर्यासते, त एव जातहर्षा गुद-
निष्क्रमणमतिवेलं कुर्वन्ति।

10

SUPERNATURAL POWERS
(GRAHABADHA)

Under Supernatural Powers (*grahabadha*) three different types of disorders may be included.

(1) Affections by supernatural powers like ghosts and witches. In these affections, manifestations of involvement of central nervous system like tremors, unconsciousness and twitching are associated with psychological symptoms like fear and laughing without reason. In addition, systemic manifestations like diarrhoea, cough and fever are also present.

Some of the entities described under *grahabadha* can be fitted under the diagnosis of heaptic coma characterised by foetor hepaticus, uraemia characterised by urine-like smell and other encephalopathies. However, one occassionally comes across cases, which do not fit with any of the known disease entities and where the aetiological factors remain idiopathic or unknown. Even today, it is not possible to disprove the existence of Supernatural powers like ghosts, witches, etc. Hence, it is important to keep in mind the possibility of affection of babies with supernatural powers and prescribe the treatment on the lines given in this chapter.

(2) Infectious diseases involving central nervous system (which in modern medicine are termed as meningitis, encephalitis, etc.) are included in Ayurveda under *grahabadha* as well as under *sannipatika jvara*.

(3) Psychiatric diseases, particularly involving disorders of personality like :

    (i) *Devagraha* (God-like personality)

    (ii) *Daityagraha* (Demon-like personality)

   (iii) *Gandharavagraha* (Engrossed in music and sex)

   (iv) *Sarpagraha* (Serpent-like personality)

   (v) *Yakshagraha* (Semi God-like personality)

   (vi) *Brahmarakshagrahas* (Demon-like personality)

   (vii) *Rakshagrahas* (Demon-like personality)

  (viii) *Pretagrahas* (Unclean person)

   (ix) *Kushmandagraha*

   (x) *Nishadagraha* (Aboriginee)

   (xi) *Ankiranagraha* (Arrogant)

   (xii) *Vetalagraha* (Sleepy personality)

  (xiii) *Pitrugraha* (Forefathers)

  (xiv) *Pishachagraha* (Ghost-like personality)

This group is characterised by the absence of organic involvement of central nervous system and systemic manifestations.

MANIFESTATIONS OF AFFECTION BY SUPERNATURAL POWERS

The premonitory symptoms are excessive crying and fever.

(i) *General Symptoms* : Fever, irritability, crying continuously, yawning, barking, screaming, shouting, biting lips, clenching teeth, clenching fists, scratching mother's as well as one's own body with nails, refusal to take feeds, miserable look, emaciation, shrill cry, excessive perspiration, excessive salivation, swelling of the eyes, conjunctivities, excessive watering of the eyes, rubbing the eyes, ears and nose, squint, vitiation of breast milk, anaemia, jaundice and palpitation are the symptoms of *graharogas*.

(ii) *Central Nervous System* : (a) *Psychological* : Fear, pulling of hair, biting the tongue and mother's breast, laughing alone without reason. (b) *Organic* : Vacant look, unconsciousness, hypotonia, drowsiness, giddiness, diminished vision, irritability, rolling of eye-balls, insotnnia, change in voice and speech, facial palsy with drooling of saliva, weak voice, jerky movements of head, paralysis, stiffness, twitching of eyelids and facial muscles, tremors, spasms of the body, opisthotonus, emprosthotonus, pleurosthotonus, fainting, ptosis, convulsions, headache, retention of urine, incontinence of urine and stool.

(iii) *Sense and Motor Organs* : Blindness, diseases of nose, ears and eyes.

(iv) *Gastro-Intestinal* : Constipation, distension, thirst, diarrhoea, vomiting, stomatitis, glossitis, borborygmi, *visuchika*. (Cholera like disease characterised by pricking pain in the abdomen).

(v) *Respiratory System* : Foam at the mouth, cough, hiccup, grunting respiration.

(vi) *Skin* : Change in colour, goose-skin, urticaria, blisters, pyoderma, perianal excoriation, prominent veins over skin of abdomen.

(vii) *Smell of the Body* : Smell of the body resembles that of fat, pus, faecal, matter, bird, crow, goat or corpse.

Smell of the Body	Affected by Graha	Characteristic Symptoms
• Fat or blood	Shanda	—
• Pus or blood	Shada Apasmara	—
• Goat or fat	Nailamesha	—
• Faeces	Shvagraha	Barking (Hydrophobia)
• Corpse	Pitru	—
• Bird	Shakuni	—
• Crow	Putana	—
• Fat or sour and foul	Shitaputana	Half of the body is cold and the other half warm
• Fish	Andhaputana	Diminished Vision
• Cow's urine or human urine	Mukhamandika	Prominent abdominal vision
• Goat	Revati	Cyanosis
• Vulture	Shushka revati	Progressive emaciation
• Foul-smelling	Lohita	—
• Vulture like and foul-smelling	Aryaka	—

Lohita, revati and *vayasi* give rise to crowing sound in the baby; *Kumari, Shakuni, Shiva, Udhvakeshi* and *Sena grahas* affect the newborn bady on 1st to 8th day respectively. Accordingly *Ravana, Nandana, Sunanda, Putana, Mukhamandika, Kathaputana, Shakunika, Sutika, Nirrhuta* and *Pilipicchika grahas* affect the babies and children on the first to eleventh day, month or year respectively. When *Revati graha* affects a girls or a lady, it leads to reproductive failure which manifests in the form of : (i) absence of secondary sex characters, (ii) absence of menstruation, (iii) abnormalities of menstruation, (iv) abortons, (v) miscarriage, (vi) fetal death, (vii) still-born badies, (viii) children dying immediately after birth, (ix) children dying within first few hours, (x) children dying within first few months, and (xi) children dying within first few years.

Some of these affected children represent cases of hereditary, congenital or metabolic diseases. The following table gives the names of various grahas and the associated conditions :

• *Shushkarevati*	Absence of menstruation and secondary sex characters
• *Katambhara*	Thin, lean and seak lady with absence of mentruation, but normal life span
• *Pushpaghni*	Normal menstruation, but sterile with presence of har on face
• *Vikrita*	The menstrual period is irregular and menstrual flow is abnormal in colour and quantity. Such a lady appears at time strong and at times very weak without any reason
• *Parisrita*	Lady becomes thin and suffers from continuous vaginal discharge
• *Andaghni*	Abortion

• *Durdhara*	Abortion with under-developed foetus whose various body parts are not differentiated
• *Kalaratri*	Miscarriage with well-developed foetus. Lady survives the miscarriage with difficulty
• *Mohini*	Lady may die during delivery
• *Stambhini*	Absence of foetal movements
• *Kroshna*	The foetus cries in uterus
• *Yapya or Dakini*	Fetal death
• *Pishachi*	Children die immediately after birth or *punyajani*
• *Pilipichhika*	Children of mothers affected by *Yakshi, Asuri, Kali, Varuni, Shashti, Bhiruka, Yamya, Matangi, Bhadrakali, Raudri, Vardhika, Chandika, Kapalamalini* and *Pilipichhika* die on second or fifteenth day
• *Vashya*	Fetal death in fifth, sixth, seventh month
• *Kulakshayakari*	Male children die but girls survive without any special effort
• *Paurushadani*	Child dies before sixteen years
• *Sandanshi*	The previous child dies when lady becomes pregnant again
• *Karkotaki*	Such as lady is afflicted with abnormal fetus, *grahas* or death
• *Indravadava*	One or both twins die
• *Vasavamukhi*	If one of the twins die, other also dies

Grahas affect the baby as they enjoy torturing or killing the baby, or for purpose of fulfilling their desires through the offering made to them by the parents of the babies. Most of the authorities feel that affection by *grahas* is a result of bad deeds of the past life of the same individual. These *grahas* do not enter the body of child themselves, but affect the babies through their innumerable, microscopic followers, which thrive on blood, fat, muscles, etc. of the baby. They thrive at night and in unclean places.

PREDISPOSING FACTORS

   (i)   Not observing cleanliness particularly after going to toilet
  (ii)   Injury or ulcers on the body
 (iii)   Not following traditions of the family
  (iv)   Non-religious conduct and cheating others
   (v)   Fear due to threatening, beating or frightening
  (vi)   Not respecting priests, saints, teachers and guests
 (vii)   Taking food in unclean and broken vessels
(viii)   Mentally unstable, selfish and greedy
  (ix)   Indulging excessively in eating, sex, sleep, exercise, harmful activities and falsehood
   (x)   Visiting lonely and inauspicious places like cemetery
  (xi)   Killing animals including cow, goat and snake

PROGNOSIS

Fatal Outcome : Continuous discharge from nose, watering of the eyes, ulcers on the tongue, grunting respiration, progressive emaciation, discolouration of skin, inability to speak, bleeding from all body orifices, burning sensation, pus-like vomitus, playing with own stools and urine, fainting off and on, stiffness, injuring self or others and entering fire or water indicate fatal outcome. Wearing fragrant flowers and ornaments, talking to ladies and young girl in lonely places, and a happy mood indicate that such a person is affected by cupid and such a person may get cured with difficulty.

Good Prognosis : Miserable, frightened and worried look, dryness of mouth, throat and lips, crying excessively, refusal to take feeds and touching the face off and on indicate good chances of recovery when affected by *graha*.

ग्रहा:

पुरा गृहस्य रक्षार्थं निर्मिता: शूलपाणिना। मनुष्यविग्रहा: पञ्च सप्त स्त्रीविग्रहा: ग्रहा:।।

स्कन्दो विशाखो मेषाख्य: श्वग्रह: पितृसंज्ञित:। शकुनी पूतना शीतपूतना-ऽदृष्टिपूतना।

मुखमण्डितिका तद्द्रेवती शुष्करेवती।।

पूर्वरूप

तेषां ग्रहीष्यतां रूपं प्रततं रोदनं ज्वर:।।

रूप

सामान्यं रूपमुत्रासजृम्भाभ्रूक्षेपदीनत:। फेनस्रावोर्ध्वदृष्ट्योष्ठदन्तदंशप्रजागरा:।।

रोदनं कूजनं स्तन्यविद्वेष: स्वरवैकृतम्। नखैरकस्मात्परित: स्वधात्र्यङ्गविलेखनम्।।

(अ. हृ. उ. 3/3-5)

असाध्य ग्रहाविष्टलक्षण

प्रस्तब्धो य: स्तनद्वेषी मुह्यते चाविशन्मुहु:।

तं बालमचिराद्धन्ति ग्रह: सम्पूर्णलक्षण:।। (सु. उ. 27/17)

साध्य ग्रहाविष्टलक्षण

विपरीतमत: साध्यं चिकित्सेदचिरार्दितम्।। (सु. उ. 27/18)

साध्य ग्रहाविष्टलक्षण

विपरीतमत: साध्यं चिकित्सेदचिरार्दितम्।। (सु. उ. 27/18)

कष्टसाध्य

रह:स्त्रीरतिसंलापगन्धस्रग्भूषणप्रिय:।।

हृष्ट: शान्तश्च दु:साध्यो रतिकामेन पीडित:। (अ. हृ. उ. 3/37)

सामान्य चिकित्सा

हन्तुकामं जयेद्धोमै: सिद्धमन्त्रप्रवर्तितै:।।

इतरौ तु यथाकामं रतिबल्यादिदानत:। (अ. हृ. उ. 3/40)

11
NATURAL CALAMITIES AND EPIDEMICS
(JANAPADODHVANSA)

A natural calamity or an epidemic may affect a region or a country involving a large number of people of different constitutions taking different diet and having different strength, resistance and digestive power. The factors that affect people in common are the wind, water, country and the season concerned. Various microbes can invade the body through the vitiated air, water or food and lead to infectious diseases.

(1) *Wind or Air* : Storms can devastate a particular region. Similarly, the air may be polluted by chemicals or bad odours, smoke, dust, moisture and sand. The air pollution predisposes to epidemics of infectious fevers, cold, cough, breathlessness, headache, vomiting and eye diseases.

(2) *Water* : Water is polluted by excreta of man and animals, chemicals, putrefying matter, bacteria, etc. Such water may have altered smell, colour, taste and temperature. If aquatic animals like fish and frogs do not survive or start leaving the reservoir, that particular reservoir should be taken as unfit for human use. Epidemics of cholera, gastro-enteritis, worm infestations, abdominal distention, fever, cough, breathlessness, cold, colicky pain, jaundice, anaemia, oedema, skin diseases, elephantiasis, gulma, heart disease, diseases of throat and head are caused by polluted water.

(3) *Region or Country* : The country may be affected by excess or inadequate rainfall or pollution by human or animal excreta, chemicals or worms. Excessive humidity in *anupa* (wet) region predisposes to *kaphaja* disorders, e.g. cough, breathlessness, oedema, tumours, etc. Wars also devastate the areas around the fronts.

(4) *Time and Season* : Abnormal season is one which has characteristics opposite to the normal season or exhibits the usual environmental changes of the season in an excessive or deficient degree. This leads to deaths due to heat stroke or subnormal temperature, etc. or predisposes to respiratory infection when exposed to heavy showers.

(5) *Infectious Diseases* : Epidemics of infectious diseases are caused by micro-organisms, when the body resistance is lowered as a result of vitiated air, water, country or season. Ayurveda mentions that these micro organisms are present all over, i. e. in earth, water and in atmosphere. They are microscopic and naturally cannot be visualised. They enter the body in large numbers, which may amount to millions. These are termed as to *jantu, sukshmakrami, Bhutas* or *rakshasas* and these *Bhutas* are supposed to be controlled by various divine powers termed as *grahas*. These micro organisms are classified as those growing on blood (*raktada*), muscles (*mansada*), fat (*vasada*), nervous tissue (*majjada*), nails (*nakhada*), teeth *(dantada)*, and *hridayachara* (those thriving on heart). They grow in unclean, moist and dark areas. They are transmitted from person to person through clothes, garlands, direct contacts, food, breath or inter-course. These are described in chapters on *krimiroga,* fever, natural calamities and epidemics, *grahabadha*, tuberculosis, ear-nose-throat-diseases, skin diseases and diseases of children in Ayurvedic texts.

Sterilisation by boiling and by exposure to various medicated fumes is advised, e.g. medicinal fumes of *guggulu, agaru, sarjarasa*, white pepper, *vacha,* salt, *nimba* (neem leaves) and ghee of goat's milk is an effective anti *bhuta* measure.

Many of the predisposing factors which lead to epidemics, e.g. atmospheric changes like excessive rain fall, low atmospheric presures, etc. are beyond human control. It is difficult to explain why a particular epidemic affects only a particular region and takes toll of lives of masses in that region. Ayurveda ascribes the epidemics to non-religious behaviour and the sinful acts of the masses. Epidemics take place when the fruits of action of the bad deeds become mature.

Treatment is divided under six caegories : (i) *Panchakarma,* i.e. Purification of body by purgative, enemas, etc. (ii) Administration of tonics, i.e. *rasayana* (iii) maintenance of high morale. This is achieved by following rules of good conduct and by worshipping God. (iv) Prevention of the epidemic or the calamity or its effects by boiling drinking water, not eating food outside, etc. (v) Treating the persons affected by appropriate measures and medicines, and (vi) As a list resort or earlier, if it is difficult to withstand its effects, one should leave the region expected to be affected by the calamity.

जनपदोध्वंस

एवमसामान्यवतामप्येभिरग्निवेश! प्रकृत्यादिभिर्भावैर्मनुष्याणां येऽन्ये भावा: सामान्यास्तद्वैगुण्यात् समानकाला: समानलिङ्गाश्च व्याधयोऽभिनिर्वर्तमाना जनपदमु-द्ध्वंसयन्ति। ते तु खल्विसे भावा: सामान्या जनपदेषु: भवन्ति।। तद्यथा-वायु:, उदकं, देश:, काल इति।   (च. वि. अ. 3/16)

तत्र वातेमेवंविविधमनारोग्यकरं विद्यात्: तद्यथा-यथर्तुविषममतिस्तिमितमतिचलमति-परुषमतिशीतमत्युष्णमतिरुक्षमत्यभिष्यन्दिनमतिभैरवारावमतिप्रतिहतपरस्परगतिमति-कुण्डलिनमसात्म्यगन्धबाष्पसिकतापांशुधूमोपहतमिति (1);

                                                                                                           (च. वि. 3)

विषौषधिपुष्पगन्धेन वायुनोपनीतेक्रम्यते यो देशस्तत्र दोषप्रकृत्यविशेषेण कासश्वा-सवमथुप्रतिश्यायशिरोरुग्ज्वरैरूपतप्यन्ते।   (सु. सू. 6/21)

धूमेऽनिले वा विषसंप्रयुक्ते, खगा: श्रमार्ता: प्रपतन्ति भूमौ कासप्रतिश्यायशिरोरुजश्च, भवन्ति तीव्रा नयनामयाश्च।।   (सु. क. 3/16, रानडे पृ. 39)

उदकं तु खल्वत्यर्थविकृतगन्धवर्णरसस्पर्श क्लेदबहुलमपक्रान्तजलचरविहङ्ग-मुपक्षीणजलेशयप्रीतिकरमपगतगुणं विद्यात् (2);   (च. वि. 3)

व्यापन्नंसलिलं यस्तु पिबतीहाप्रसाधितम्।

श्वयथुं पाण्डुरोगश्च त्वग्दोषमविपाकताम्।।

श्वासकासप्रतिश्यायशूलगुल्मोदराणि च ।

अन्यानवा विषमान् रोगान् प्राप्नुयादचिरेण स: । (सु. सू. 45/16)

"स्थिरा: (नद्य:) कृमि-श्लीपद-हृत् कंठ शिरोरोगान्प्रकुर्वते" ।

(अ. हृ. सू. 5/10)

तासामुपयोगाद्द्विविधरोगप्रादुर्भावो मरको वा भवेदिति । (सु. सू. 6/19)

देशं पुन: प्रकृतिविकृतवर्णगन्धरसस्पर्शं क्लेदबहुलमुपसृष्टं सरीसृपव्यालमशकशलभ-मक्षिकामूषकोलूककश्माशानिकशकुनिजम्बुकादिभिस्तृणोलूपोपवनवन्तं प्रतानादिबहुल-मपूर्ववदवपतिततशुष्कनष्टशस्यं धूम्रपवनं प्रध्मातपत्त्रिगणमुत्क्रुष्टश्वगणमुद्भ्रान्त-व्यथितविविधमृगपक्षिसङ्घमुत्सृष्टनष्टधर्मसत्यलज्जाचारशीलगुणजनपदं शश्वत्क्षु-भितोदीर्णसलिलाशयं प्रततोल्कापातनिर्घातभूमिकम्पमतिभयारावरूपं रुक्षताम्रारुणसि-ताभ्रजालसंवृतार्कचन्द्रतारकमभीक्ष्णं ससम्भ्रमोद्वेगमिव सत्रासरुदितमिव सतमस्कमिव गुह्यकाचरितमिवाक्रन्दितशब्दबहुलं चाहितं विद्यात् (3);

(च. वि. 3)

तथा शस्त्रप्रभवस्यापि जनपदोद्ध्वंसस्याधर्म एव हेतुर्भवति । येऽतिप्रवृद्धलोभक्रोध-मोहमानास्ते दुर्बलानवमत्यात्मस्वजनपरोपघाताय शस्त्रेण परस्परमभिक्रामन्ति, परान् वाऽभिक्रामन्ति परैर्वाऽभिक्राम्यन्ते ।।

(च. वि. 3)

जाङ्गल-आनुपदेशा:

जाङ्गलं वातभूयिष्ठमानूपं तु कफोल्बणम् ।। (अ. हृ. सू. 1/23)

कालं तु खलु यथर्तुलिङ्गाद् विपरीतलिङ्गं मतिलिङ्गं हीनलिङ्गं चाहितं व्यवस्येत् (4);

(च. वि. 3)

भूता: जन्तव:

रक्षोगणादिभिर्वा विविधैर्भूतसङ्घैस्तमधर्ममन्यद् वाऽप्यपचारान्तरमुपलभ्याभिहन्यन्ते ।।

(च. वि. 3/22)

पृथिव्यामन्तरीक्षे च ये चरन्ति निशाचरा: ।

दिक्षु वास्तुनिवासाश्च पान्तु त्वां ते नमस्कृता: । (सु. सू. 5/22)

योन्यामधावनात् कण्डूं जाता: कुर्वन्ति जन्तव: ।

सा स्यादचरणा कण्डूवा तयाऽतिनरकाङ्क्षिणी । (च. चि. 30/18)

न ते मनुष्यै: सह संविशन्ति न वा मनुष्यान् क्वचिदाविशन्ति ।

ये त्वाविशन्तीति वदन्ति मोहात् ते भूतविद्याविषयादपोह्या:।।

तेषां ग्रहाणां परिचारका ये कोटीसहस्रायुतपद्यसंख्या:।

असृग्वसामांसभुज: सुभीमा निशाविहाराश्च तमाविशन्ति।।

(सु. उ. 60/22–23)

ओजोशनानां रजनीचराणामाहारहेतोर्न शरीरमिष्टम्।

गर्भं हरेयुर्यदि ते न मातुर्लब्धावकाशा न हरेयुरोज:।।   (च. शा. 2/10)

प्रसङ्गात्गात्रसंस्पर्शान्ति:श्वासात् सहभोजनात्।

एकशय्यासनाच्चैव वस्त्रमाल्यानुलेपनात्।

कुष्ठं ज्वरश्च शोषश्च नेत्राभिष्यन्द एव च।

औपसर्गिकिरोगाश्च संक्रामन्ति नरान्नरम्।

(मा. नि. कुष्ठनिदान 42, 43, पृ. 343)

दर्पणादीन् यथा छाया शीतोष्णं प्राणिनो यथा।

विशन्ति न च दृश्यन्ते ग्रहास्तद्वच्छरीरिणाम्।   (सु. उ. 60/19–20)

ततो गुग्गुल्वगुरुसर्जरसवचागौरसर्षपचूर्णैर्लवणनिम्बपत्रविमिश्रैराज्ययुक्तैर्धूपयेत्।

(सु. सू. 5/18)

वैगुण्यमुपन्नानां देशकालनिलाम्भसाम्। गरीयस्त्वं विशेषेण हेतुमत् संप्रवक्ष्यते।।

वाताज्जलं जालादेशं देशात् कालं स्वभावत:। विद्यात् दुष्परिहार्यत्वाद-

गरीयस्तरमर्थवित्।।   (च. वि. 3/9–10)

येषां न मृत्युसामान्यं सामान्यं न कर्मणाम्।

कर्म पञ्चविधं तेषां भेषजं परमुच्यते।।   (च. वि. 3/13)

रसायनानां विधिवच्चोपयोग: प्रशस्यते। शस्यते देहवृत्तिश्च भेषजै: पूर्वमुद्धतै:।।

सत्यं भूते दया दानं बलयो देवतार्चनम्। सद्वृत्तस्यानुवृत्तिश्च प्रशमो गुप्तिरात्मन:।।

हितं जनपदानां च शिवानामुपसेवनम्। सेवनं ब्रह्मचर्यस्य तथैव ब्रह्मचारिणाम्।।

सङ्कथा धर्मशास्त्राणां महर्षीणां जितात्मनाम्। धार्मिकै: सात्त्विकैर्नित्यं सहास्या

वृद्धसम्मतै:।।

इत्येद् भेषजं प्रोक्तामायुष: परिपालनम्। येषामनियतो मृत्युस्तस्मिन् काले सुदारुणे।।

(च. वि. 3/14–20)

वाय्वादीनां यद्वैगुण्यमुत्पद्यते तस्य मूलमधर्म:, तन्मूलं वाऽसत्कर्म पूर्वकृतं; तयोर्योनि:

प्रज्ञापराध एव।

(च. वि. 3)

12

PATHOGENESIS
(SAMPRAPTI VIJNYANAM)

Health is defined as a balanced state, while disease represents unbalanced state of *doshas* (*Vata, Pitta* and *Kapha), dhatus* (tissues) and *mala* (waste products). The deviation from robust health to diseased state is brought about by the aetiological factors, which increase or decrease or vitiate the *doshas, dhauts* and *mala.* Hereditary factors like constitution, etc. predispose to a particular group of disease, which become manifest by the action of environmental seasonal and dietary factors, weak digestive power, etc. as well as other unknown factors, which give rise to imbalance in the state of *doshas.* It is this imbalanced state of *doshas,* which give rise to diseased state. Person with good defence mechanism of the body (*vyadhisahatva*) with good quality of digestive and tissue enzymes may by able to digest the *doshas* and ward off further increase and accomulation of *doshas* by following appropriate do's and don'ts as far diet and activities are concerned.

Quality of mind depends on the dominance of particle of *raja, tama* or *sattva* their balance state. As far as mind is concerned, *rajasika* and *tamasik* personalities are considered to be diseased ones, where as *sattvik* is considered to be healthy and highly evolved mental state, which is superseded only by *trigunatit* personality. Details of these are described in the first part of basic principles of Ayurveda. As described there, their qualities are dependant on the fine *raja, tama* and *sattva* qualities.

Pathogenesis gives the insight into the development of the disease. It gives us an exact idea as to how the aetiological factors gives rise to increased formation of *doshas,* how the *doshas* travel at different sites setting in the disease process. The development of the disease is described under six stages, viz. *chaya, prakopa, prasara, sthanasanshraya, vyakti* and *bheda*.

ACCUMULATION OF DOSHAS (CHAYA STAGE)

When the aetiological factors are not powerful, the *doshas* accumulate slowly and in small amounts, e.g. the increased *Vata dosha* produced by the dryness and lightness of the air in *grishma*, i.e. summer is partially subduced by the heat of *grishma*. Hence, *Vata dosha* accumulates only to a limited extent, i.e. in small amount in the body and is is termed as *Vata-chaya*. Similarly, accumulation to a limited extent of *Pitta* and *Kapha dosha*, i.e. *Pitta chaya* and *Kapha dosha,* occurs in *varsha*, i.e. rainy season and *shishir,* i.e. winter season respectively.

The *doshas* tend to collect locally depending on the aetiological factors, e.g. dietetic indiscretion, excessive activity and breathing moist air would result in accumulation of *doshas* in gastro-intestinal tract, muscles and lungs respectively. *Doshas* also collect in their specific sites, e. g. *doshas* due to dietetic indiscretion tend to collect in colon, small intestine an stomach in *Vata, Pitta* and *Kapha chayas* respectively.

Clinical Manifestations : The clinical manifestations are fullness of stomach in *Vata chaya,* yellowish discoloration of skin in *Pitta chaya* and weak digestive power, heaviness of body and laziness in *Kapha chaya.* In addition, one develops aversion to the aetiological factor, e.g. if one takes excess of cold drinks and *Vata chaya* occurs, one develops aversion to cold drinks. If *Vata chaya* occurs due to eating in excess dry food items, one develops aversion to dry food items.

Course : The accumulated *doshas* may come back to normal level or may increase and lead to second stage of *prakopa*. Sometimes *doshas* lie dormant in one stage for a long time till additional causative or precipitating factors stimulate them when they progress to next stage.

Natural Cure for the Accumulated Doshas : The diurnal variations which lead to accumulation of *doshas* tend to correct increased *doshas* themselves, e.g. increased *Kapha* in the morning comes to normal level by the heat in the afternoon.

Development of aversions to the aetiological factors in *chaya* stage also tend to correct the increased *dosha*, e.g. eating excess of sweets leads to accumulation of *Kapha dosha*. This gives rise to aversion to sweets, which in turn results in natural cure.

The accumulated *dosha* may remain dormant for some time and later lead to *prakopa* stage when triggered by dietetic or environmental factors, e.g. *Vata chaya* in *grishma* season results in *Vata prakopa* in *varsha* season due to cold environment.

Chaya stage will quickly lead to *prakopa* stage, if aetiological factors are powerful or one does not pay attention to the natural caution signal, i.e. aversion to the aetiological factors.

Treatment : It is important to threat the *doshas* in *chaya* stage, as they constitute the seeds of disease, which should not be allowed to germinate.

The treatment consists of avoiding aetiological factors, which would be indicated by development of natural aversion to them. In addition, one should neutralise the increased *dosha* by appropriate treatment, i.e. by *langhana*, if *dosha* is in small amounts, by *dipana* and *prachana*, if *doshas* are in moderate quantity and getting rid of *doshas* by emesis, purgatives or enemas if *doshas* are in large quantity.

ACCUMULATION OF DOSHAS İN EXCESS (PRAKOPA STAGE)

When aetiological factors are not controlled and continue to act for long the *doshas* continue to increase further and accumulate in excess till they reach the *prakopa* stage.

Clinical Manifestation : Pain in abdomen and awareness of movements of gases in abdomen occur in *Vata prakopa*. *Pitta prakopa* gives rise to thirst, regurgitation with sour taste and burning sensation. Nausea and disgust for food are the symptoms of *Kapha prakopa*. In addition, one develops a desire for factors and substances having properties opposite to the causative agents. This desire is obvious, when a single powerful factor is acting for quite sometime and may not be seen when multiple factors are operating.

Course : As in *chaya* stage, the *doshas* in *prakopa* stage may subside naturally, when the season changes. If appropriate action is taken the *doshas* will subside quickly. The *doshas* may remain dormant for sometime and get reactivated, when aetiological or precipitating factor trigger them. When the aetiological factors are powerful and or continue to act for quite sometime. The *doshas* will further increase and may lead to third stage of *prasara*.

Treatment : Treatment consists of administering substances having properties opposite to those of aetiological factors.

DISSEMINATION OF DOSHAS (PRASARA STAGE)

Prasara stage means stage of dissemination of *doshas*. When one or more factors responsible for a particular disease continue to further excite the *dosha* which are already in the *prakopa* stage the *doshas* disseminate in the bod, This is termed as *prasara* stage. The dissemination of the *doshas* of *prasara* stage is compared to the over flow from a vessel full of flour, which is undergoing fermentation. *Vata dhatu* which is responsible for all the movements the body including movements of body fluids is also responsible for the dissemination of the accumulated *Vata, Pitta* and *Kapha doshas* from the local sites. Depending upon the aetiological factors, the three *doshas* may accumulat singly or in various combination and get disseminated through body fluids or blood.

Clinical Manifestations : Pain due to movements of *Vata* in abnormal direction and gurgling noise in abdomen are the symptoms of *Vata prasara*. Localised burning pain simulating that due to sucking, burning sensation all over the body and sensation as if body is full of smoke are the symptoms of *Pitta prasara.* *Kapha prasara* gives rise to anorexia, vomiting, indigestion and a state of exhaustion.

Compared to the previous two stages, the symptoms are more generalised during this stage. The person will develop desires, which will try to neutralise the disseminated *doshas* in all possible manners.

Course : As in the stage of *prakopa*, the disseminated *doshas* may subside or remain dormant for some time and get reactivated again or increase further and lead to the next stage of *sthanasanshraya*.

Treatment : The treatment consists of neutralising the increased or vitiated *doshas* or by all possible means.

Till this stage, the body tissues or organs are not involved and the treatment is directed towards normalisation of affected *dosha* or *doshas*.

LOCALISATION OF DOSHAS (STHANASANSHRAYA STAGE)

This is a stage of localisation of disseminated *doshas* in a particular site or stage of prodromal symptoms. The disseminated *doshas* get localised in a tissue or organ whose defence mechanism is weak. The poor local defence mechanism may be genetic or acquired. The aquired cause may be dietetic, environmental, traumatic or sequelae of previous illness, etc. Though in the disseminated stage of *prasara*, the *doshas* are present all over the body, their concentration in any tissue or organ is not much. In addition, the *doshas* in *prasara* stage, though in superficial contact, do not enter or affect the individual cells of any organ. On the other hand, in the stage of *sthanasanshraya*, the concentration of *doshas* in a particular organ is much more. During this stage, the *doshas* enter the individual cells of the tissue or organ and cause their slight dysfunction.

Vata, Pitta and *Kapha* are the three basic biological elements which constitute the bodies of all the living creatures. Each cell and organ though composed of all the three elements has one dominant biological element, e.g. *Pitta* dominates in small intestine, *Kapha* in lungs and *Vata* in ears. When the causative *dosha* gets localised and enters the cells of the organ, it disturbs the balance of *Vata, Pitta* and *Kapha* in that organ.

The dominant biological element in particular organ naturally is offended to the maximum extent and now becomes local *dosha*, i.e. local *Vata, Pitta* and *Kapha dosha*. This results in dysfunction of organ involved. In generalised diseases like fever (septicemias) there is no specific localisation of causative *doshas* in a particular organ but they get localised in and affect all the cells and tissues of the body.

Clinical Manifestation : During the stage of *chaya, prakopa* and *prasara,* the manifestations are non-specific and are related to the increased or vitiated *dosha.* In the stage of *sthanasanshraya* one gets premonitory or prodromal symptoms of a disease which depend on slight affection of the involved organ or tissue as well as the causative *dosha.* These premonitory symptoms are usually described under individual diseases. During this stage, the patient develops aversion for substances and factors which would further increase or vitiate the local as well as the causative *dosha.*

Course : In this stage, *doshas* may damage the tissue or organ further till the disease manifests, i.e. *vyakta* stage, or the tissue might recover completely from the local imbalance of the *doshas.*

Treatment : The principle of treatment consists of treating the local *dosha* simultaneously keeping in mind that the causative *dosha* is not aggravated, e.g. in *sthansashraya* stage of cough caused by *Pitta dosha,* one should treat the local *Kapha dosha,* simultaneously seeing that at the same time the causative *Pitta dosha* does not increase. Occasionally if the causative *dosha* is very powerful, one should treat the causative *dosha* simultaneously seeing that the local *dosha* does not increase.

PREMONITORY SYMPTOMS (PURVA-RUPA)

Premonitory symptoms represent all the signs an symptoms

which are observed before the manifestations of the disease appear. These symptoms may appear during the stage of accumulation (*Chaya*), increase (*Prakopa*), spread (*Prasara*) or localisation of the *doshas* in the tissue or organ (*Sthanasan-shraya*). The premonitory symptoms represent the resistance offered by the tissue or the organs to the attacking *doshas*. Whereas the manifestations of the disease means that the diseased tissue or the organs are now overpowered by the *doshas*.

The premonitory symptoms are classified as general and specific premonitory symptoms. They are related to the *dosha* which is increased in that disease. If all the prodromal symptoms described in a disease are present, it takes a fatal course.

It is important to start the treatment in prodromal stage, as given in the chapter on stages of the disease, i.e. *Chaya-prakopa,* e.g. during prodromal stage of fever, fasting or light diet is advised. However, during prodromal stage of *vataja* fever, administration of ghee is indicated, so that the disease is either subdued or takes a milder form, if it becomes manifest.

DISEASE STAGE (VYAKTA STAGE)

When the causative *doshas* accumulate in excess and cause significant damage to the tissues or organ, the disease manifests itsele The classical symptoms and signs of the disease now become apparent. The clinical manifestation depends on the organ involved as well as the causative *dosha*. They are described under individual diseases in standard text books.

Clinical Manifestations of Disease, i.e. Rupa : *Rupa, linga, lakshana, chinnha, akriti, vyanjana* and *sansthana* are equivalents and are used synonymously. These are related to the affected *doshas* as well as the organ or the tissue. The symptoms arise as a result of increase, decrease or vitiation of *dosha*. The same symptoms are termed as clinical manifestation of disease, if it arises as a result of damage to a tissue or organ by *dosha*. A person with good resisting power, even when afflicted with a major disease, appear to be suffering from a minor disease and vice-versa.

The clinical manifestations as well as prodromal symptoms indicates the *doshas*, tissue or the organ affected in a disease, e.g. colicky pain, burning sensation and sensation of heaviness indicate increase in *Vata*, *Pitta* and *Kapha* respectively. Pallor, cramps in muscles, emaciation and pain in the bones indicate affection of blood, mucular tissue, fatty tissue and bony tissue respectively. Cough, diarrhoea and unconsciousness indicate the affection of respiratory, gastro-intestinal and nervous system respectively.

The clinical manifestations give us an important clue to the diagnosis, the stage of the disease, differential diagnosis, prognosis and treatment in every case. In Ayurveda, diseases are often named after the most important or the main symptom, e.g. *kasa*, i.e. cough can be a symptom of many disease or it may be a disease entity itself, e.g. cough is a symptom of heart disease or hysteria, while when one talks of *kasa* as a disease entity, one has tracheo-bronchitis in the mind.

In practice, majority of the patients seek the advice of physician for one or two symptoms like headache, burning sensation, etc. In many of these cases, one does not find any evidence of affection of tissues or organs. Hence, these persons cannot be labelled as suffering from a particular disease. Detection and correction of the root cause and treatment to correct the unbalanced state of *doshas* is enough to cure the symptom. On the other hand, when a person suffers from disease entity, apart from correcting the causative factors and *doshas*, one has to protect and increase the resistance of the tissue and organ attacked by *doshas*. Hence, symptoms can be easily controlled, while the disease entity takes longer time to settle. In addition, it is important to follow do's and don'ts during convalescence and afterwards also till normal state of tissues and organs is restored.

STAGE OF BHEDA

It is the stage of differentiation of the type of disease. During this stage, if the disease is localised superficially as in an abscess, the pus comes out by rupture of the abscess and the body gets rid off the *doshas* and the damaged tissues. In diseases like fever, the body cannot get rid off the *doshas* quickly. Hence such diseases tend to become chronic. During this stage, these differentiate furth depending on the particular *doshas* affected, e.g. *Vataja* fever *Pittaja* fever, *Kaphaja* fever, etc. If not treated properly and in time, they may become chronic or incurable.

The various stages of pathogenesis have been summarised in the table page No. 125.

UPADRAVA (COMPLICATION)

Complication is a separate disease, which arises during or immediatetly after the course of an existing disease and which is dependent on the existence, of the original or main disease. The original disease acts as one of the important cause of the complication. The lowered resistance of the patient during the course of the original disease acts as a predisposing factor for the development of its complication.

CAUSES OF COMPLICATIONS

(i) Aetiological factors continue to act and lead to formation, accumulation and spread of *doshas* which affect and settle in other organs of the body giving rise to complication, e.g. germs of pneumonia settling in brain and giving rise to brain abscess.

(ii) Increased *doshas* which act as aetiological factors of original disease are further increased because if the patient does not follow the instructions regading diet and activity, e.g. a patient with pneumonia develops empyema because he takes cold drinks and ice-cream and uses air-conditioned room.

(iii) In addition, when different aetiological factors operate during the course of existing disease, they can also lead to development of complication. Here the *doshas* responsible for the original disease and its complication are not identical. In some cases, the patient is completely, cured of the original disease, while its complication persists after it, e.g. patient with measles develops bronchopneumonia due to germs of pneumonia settling in the lungs. Here the raw area in the lungs caused measles virus acts as a predisposing factor.

When a patient develops new symptoms or clinical manifestations, it is important to differentiate between development of a complication and occurence of new disease entity. The aetiological factors, causative *doshas* and pathogenesis are same as those of the original disease or the original disease is related to the complication, as it acts as a predisposing factor for development of the complications. On the other hand the aetiological factors, causative *doshas* and pathogenesis are different when a new disease is superimposed on the first disease. In addition, two diseases are in way related to each other, e.g. patient with measles develops chickenpox or mumps.

How can we differentiate between stage of a disease and a complication? When a disease progresses, new clinical manifestations are encountered depending on the stage of the disease, e.g. in small pox one gets stages of papules, vesicles, pustules and scab formation. Similarly, in many diseases, we get *Samavastha* followed by *nirama avastha*. Though the clinical manifestations may vary from stage to stage, the site of the disease remains the same in all the stages. On the other hand, in complications the disease affects a site different from the original site of the disease. Sometimes the complication may occur at the same site as the original disease. However, the character of the lesion and the manifestations are quite different from those described under various stages of the same disease, e.g. development of secoudary infection in the form of boils and abscess in a case of scabies.

PATHOGENESIS

	Chaya stage	Prakopa	Prasara	Sthanasanshraya	Vyakta	Bheda
• Dosha	+ (Local)	++ (Local)	+++ (Dissemination)	+ Localisation in an organ	++ Damage to the organ	+++ Damage to the organ. Further differentiation of type of *dosha* e.g. *Vataja, Pittaja, Kaphaja*
• Vata	Fullness of stomach	Pain in abdomen, consciousness of gaseous movements with in abdomen	Pain all over the body, gurgling noises in abdomen	Vary with disease or organ involved	Clinical manifestations of disease	
• Pitta	Yellowish discolouration of skin	Thirst, acid regurgitation, burning sensation	Burning and smoky sensation all over body			
• Kapha	Heaviness of body and laziness	Nausea, disgust	Anorexia, vomiting, exhaustion			
• General	Aversion to aetiological facrots, e.g. cold drinks	Desire for factors and substances having opposite properties, e.g. hot drinks	Aversion for causative factors and desire for opposite factors			
• Phase in modern medicine	Incubation period	incubation period	Dissemination (a) Rapid, e.g. spticemia (b) Slow	Prodromal phase with premonitory Symptoms	Clinical manifestations	Type of disease or stage of disease well-differentiated

Apart from these stages, pathogenesis is also described under *Sankhya Vikalpa, Pradhanya, Bala* and *Kala.*

(i) *Sankhya Samprapti* : Each disease is classified into different sub-types, e.g. *jvara*, i.e. fever is classified into eight varieties, *kasa*, i.e. cough is classified into five sub-types. It is important to know exact number, i.e. varieties of disease entity so that one can get complete idea of disease process.

(ii) *Vikalpa Samprapti* : It is not enough to know which *dosha* is affected. It is important that the physician takes into consideration the degree to which each *dosha* is increased, decreased or vitiated. This concept of the extent to which each *dosha* is increased, decreased vitiated, the exact and relative state of each *dosha* is known as, *vikalpa samprapti.*

(iii) *Pradhana Samprapti* : In a particular disease, many causative factors may be at work and may give rise to the disease in different ways. It is important to know *pradhana*, i.e. the most important cause and the most important mechanism of the development of the disease.

(iv) *Bala Samprapti* : It is important to know *bala*, i.e. how powerful or strong are the causative factors, *doshas*, premonitory symptoms, clinical manifestations, etc.

(v) *Kala Samprapti* : The relation of time of the day, night as well as the season of onset, aggravation and relief of the disease is termed as *kala samprapti* and gives important clue to the causative *dosha.*

संप्राप्ति विज्ञानम्

प्रस्तावना

विकारो धातुवैषम्यं साम्यं प्रकृतिरुच्यते ।   (च. सू. 9/4)

रोगस्तु दोषवैषम्यं, दोषसाम्यमरोगता ।   (अ. ह. सू. 1/20)

काल: परिणाम:

परिणाम: अयोगादियुक्ता ऋतुस्वभावजा शीतादया: ।   (मा. नि. टी. 8)

काल: पुन: परिणाम उच्यते, कालोऽहि सर्वं परिमयति इति अत: परिणाम:।

निर्दिष्ट कालसम्प्राप्ति: व्याधीनां व्याधिसंग्रहे। चयप्रकोपप्रशमा: पित्तादीनां यथा पुरा।।

मिथ्यातिहीनलिङ्गाश्च वर्षान्ता रोगहेतव:। जीर्णभुक्तप्रजीर्णान्नकालाकालस्थितिश्च या।

पूर्वमध्यापराह्णाश्च रात्र्या यामास्त्रयश्च ये। एषु कालेषु नियता ये रोगास्ते च कालजा:।।
(च. शा. 1/110, 112)

कालस्य परिणामेन जरामृत्युनिमित्तजा:।

रोगा: स्वभाविका: दृष्ट: स्वभावो निष्प्रतिक्रिया:।। (च. शा. 1/115)

चयप्रकोपप्रशमा: वायोर्ग्रीष्मादिषु त्रिषु।

वर्षादिषु तु पित्तस्य, श्लेष्मण: शिशिरादिषु।।

वयोऽहोरात्रिभुक्तानां तेऽन्तमध्यादिग: क्रमात्। (अ. हृ. सू. 9/4)

दैवम्

निर्निष्टं दैवशब्देन कर्म यत् पौर्वदेहिकम्। हेतुस्तदपि कालेन रोगाणामुपलभ्यते।।

न हि कर्म महत् किञ्चित् फलं यस्य न भुज्यते। (च. शा. 1/116)

दैवमात्मकृतं विद्यात् कर्म यत् पौर्वदेहिकम्।

स्मृत: पुरुषकारस्तु क्रियते यदिहापरम्।। (च. वि. 3/30)

युगे युगे धर्मपाद: क्रमेणपानेन हीयते।

गुणपादश्च भूतानामे वं लोक: प्रलीयते।।

संवत्सरशते पूर्णे याति संवत्सर: क्षयम्।

देहिनामायुष: काले यम यन्मानमिष्यते।।

इति विकाराणां प्रागुत्पत्तिहेतुस्क्तो भवति। (च. वि. 3/25, 26, 27)

चयावस्था

चयो वृद्धि: स्वाधम्न्येव प्रद्वेषो वृद्धिहेतुषु। (अ. हृ. सू. 12/22)

स्वस्थानवृद्धिर्दोषाणां चय इत्यभिधीयते।

ग्रीष्मे वातचय:

चीयते लघुरुक्षाभिरेषधीभि: समीरण:। तद्विधस्तद्विधे देहे कालस्यौष्ण्यान्न कुप्यति।।

वर्षायां पित्तचय:

अद्भिरम्लविपाकाभिरेषधीभिश्च तादृशम्। पित्तं याति चयं कोपं न तु कालस्य शैत्यत:।।

शिशिरे कुफचय:

चीयते स्निग्धशीताभिरुदकौषधिभि: कफ:। तुल्येऽपि काले देहे च स्कन्नत्वान्
प्रकुप्यति।।   (अ. हृ. सू. 12/25, 26, 27)

चयलक्षणानि

तत्र संचितानां खलु दोषाणां स्तब्धपूर्णकोष्ठता पीतावभासता मन्दोष्मता चाङ्गाना
गौरवं चयकारणविद्वेष: चेति लिंगानि भवन्ति। एष प्रथमक्रियान्काल:।

चायवस्थे उपचार:

चायदीन् यान्ति सद्योऽपि दोषा: कालेऽपि वा न तु।   (अ. हृ. सू. 12/28)
चय एवं जयेद्दोषं कुपितं त्वविरोधयन्।
तत्र प्रथम: क्रियाकाल:।   (अ. हृ. सू. 32–15; सु. सू. 21/18)
तत्रस्थाश्च विलम्बेरन् भूयो हेतुप्रतीक्षिण:।
ते कालादिबलं लब्ध्वा कुप्यन्त्यन्याश्रयेष्वपि।।   (अ. हृ. सू. 13/19)
सञ्चयेऽपहता दोषा लभन्ते नोत्तरा गती:।
ते तूतरासु गतिषु भवन्ति बलवत्तरा:।।   (सु. सू. 22/37)
तत्राल्पे लङ्घनं पथ्यं, मध्ये लङ्घनपाचनम्।
प्रभूते शोधनं, तद्धि मूलादुन्मूलयेन्मलान्।।   (अ. हृ. सू. 8/21)

दोषप्रकोपलक्षणानि

तेषां प्रकोपात् कोष्ठतोदसञ्चरणाम्लिकापिपासापरिदाहान्नद्वेषहृदयोत्क्लेदाश्च जायन्ते।
तत्र द्वितीय क्रियाकाल:।   (सु. सू. 21/27)

प्रकोप:

वृद्धिर्हि द्विधा चयप्रकोपभेदेन।   (अ. सं.)
चयो वृद्धि: स्वधाम्न्येव कोपस्तून्मार्गगामिता।   (अ. हृ. सू.)
देहेऽतिरूपा वृद्धिश्चय: विलयनरूपा वृद्धि: प्रकोप:।   (डल्हण)

प्रकोपे चिकित्सा

चय एव जयेद्दोषं कुपितं त्वविरोधयन्।
सर्वकोपे बलीयांसं शेषदोषविरोधत:।।   (अ. हृ. सू. 12/15)

प्रसर:

अत ऊर्ध्वं प्रसरं वक्ष्याम:–तेषामेभिराङ्खविशेषै: प्रकुपितानां पर्युषितकिण्वोद-

कपिष्टसमवाय इवोद्रिक्तानां, प्रसरो भवति। तेषां वायुर्गतिमत्त्वात् प्रसरणहेतु:
सत्यप्यचैतन्ये। स हि रजोभूयिष्ठ:, रजश्च प्रवर्त्तकं सर्वभावानाम्। यथा–महानुद-
कसञ्चयोऽतिवृद्ध: सेतुमवदार्याेपरेणोदकेन व्यामिश्र: सर्वत: प्रधावति। एवं दोषा:
कदाचिदेकशों द्विश: समस्ता: शोणितसहिता व अनेकधा प्रसरन्ति। तद्यथा–वात:,
पित्तम्, श्लेष्मा, शोणितम्, वातपित्ते, वातश्लेष्माणौ, वातशोणिते, पित्तशोणिते,
श्लेष्मशोणिते, वातपित्तशोणितानि, वातश्लेष्मशोणितानि, पित्तश्लेष्मशोणितानि,
वातापित्तकफा:, वातपित्तकफशोणितानि; इत्येवं पञ्चदशधा प्रसरन्ति।।

कृत्स्नेऽर्द्धेऽवयवे वाऽपि यत्राङ्गे कुपितो भृशम्। दोषो विकारं नभसि मेघवत्तत्र
वर्पति।।

नात्यर्थं कुपितश्चापि लीनो मार्गे तिष्ठति।

निष्प्रत्यलीक: कालेन हेतुमासाद्य कुप्यति।। (सु. सू. 21/28–30)

प्रसरस्य लक्षणानि

एवं प्रकुपितानां प्रसरतां च वायोर्विमार्गगमनाततोपौ, ओषचोषपरिदाहधूमायनानि
पित्तस्य, अरोचकाविपाकाङ्गसादाच्छर्दिर्देशचेति श्लेष्मणो लिङ्गानि भवन्ति।

तत्र तृतीय: क्रियाकाल:। (सु. सू. 21/32)

प्रसरे चिकित्सा

तत्र प्रसरं यावद्दोषाणां एव हेतुलिङ्ग चिकित्सा तदनन्तरं व्याधेरिति।

(सु. सू. 21/38 टीका)

स्थानसंश्रय:

अत ऊर्ध्वं स्थानसंश्रयं वक्ष्याम: एवं प्रकुपिता: तास्तान् शरीरप्रदेशानागम्य तांस्तान्
व्याधीन् जनयन्ति। ते यदोदरसन्निवेशं कुर्वन्ति तदा गुल्मविद्रध्युराग्निसङ्गऽनाह
विसूचिकाऽतिसारप्रभृतीन् जनयन्ति। बस्तिगता: प्रमेहाश्मरीमूत्राघातमूत्रदोषप्रभृतीन्।
वृषणगता वृद्धि: मेढ्रगता निरुद्धप्रकशपदंशशूकदोषप्रभृतीन्। गुदगता भगन्दराशो:
प्रभृतीन्। ऊर्ध्वजत्रुगतास्तूर्ध्वजान्। त्वङ्मांसशोणितस्था: क्षुद्ररोगान् कुष्ठानि विस-
पाँश्च। मेदोगता ग्रन्थ्यपच्यर्बुदगण्डालजीप्रभृतीन्, अस्थिगता विद्रध्यनुश-
यीप्रभृतीन्। पादगता: श्लीपदवातशोणितवातकण्टकप्रभृतीन्, सर्वाङ्गगताज्वरसर्वाङ्ग
रोगप्रभृतीन्। तेषामेवभिनिविष्टानां पूर्वरूप प्रादुर्भाव:, तं प्रतिरोगं वक्ष्याम:। तत्र
पूर्वरूपगतेषु चतुर्थ क्रियाकाल:। चिकित्साचात्र दोषस्य चेत्युभयाश्रिता।

(सु. सू. 21/ 33)

कुपितानां हि दोषाणां शरीरे परिधावताम्।। (सु. सू. 24/19)

खवैगुण्यात्-स्रोतोवैगुण्यात् इत्यर्थ:।

स्थानसञ्चय: दोषदूष्यस्थ संश्रय:।   (चक्रदत्त टीका 21/33)

स्थानसंश्रय लक्षणानि

स्थानसंश्रयिण: क्रुद्धा भाविव्याधिप्रबोधकम्। दोषा: कुर्वन्ति यल्लिङ्गं पूर्वरूपं तदुच्यते।।

व्याधि दर्शनम्-व्यक्ति:

अत ऊर्ध्व व्याधेर्दर्शनं वक्ष्याम:–

शोफार्बुदग्रन्थिविद्रधिविसर्पप्रभृतीनां प्रव्यक्त, लक्षणता, ज्वरातिसारप्रभृतीनाञ्च। तत्र पञ्चम: क्रियाकाल:।।   (सु. सू. 21/34)

भेद:

अत ऊर्ध्व मेतेषामेवदीर्णानां व्रणभावमापन्नानां षष्ठ: क्रियाकाल:। ज्वरातिसार-प्रभृतीनाश्च दीर्घकालानुबन्ध:। तत्राप्रतिक्रियमाणेऽसाध्यतामुपयान्ति।

(सु. सू. 21/35)

उपद्रव:

उपद्रवति, उत्पद्यमानस्यव्याधे: समीपे उपैतीत्युपद्रव:, उपद्रवस्य व्याधे: पश्चाज्जायमानत्वात्।

उपद्रवस्तु खलु रोगोत्तरकालजो रोगाश्रयो रोग एव स्थूलोऽणुर्वा, रोगात् पश्चाज्जायत इत्युपद्रवसंज्ञ:। तत्र प्रधानो व्याधि:।

व्याधेर्येगुणभूत उपद्रवतस्य प्राय: प्रधानप्रशमे प्रशमो भवति। स तु पीडाकरतरे भवति।

पश्चादुत्पद्यमानो व्याधिपरिक्लिष्टशरीरत्वात्। तस्मादुपद्रवं त्वरमाणोऽभिबाधेत।

(च. चि. 21/40)

व्याधेरूपरियोव्याधिर्भक्त्युत्तकालज:। उपक्रमावियोधीच स उपद्रव उच्यते।।

(सु. उ. 39/290)

पूर्वोद्भवनिमित्तेन योऽपरो जायते गद:। तमुपद्रवमित्याहु: अतीसारो यथा ज्वरे।।

(का. सू. 27/57)

13

SYMPTOMS AND THEIR SIGNIFICANCE
(ROGALAKSHANANI TESHAM MAHATVAM CHA)

Every symptom arises as a result of (1) Imbalance of *doshas,* i.e. *Vata, Pitta* and *Kapha.* (2) Increased, decreased or vitiated state of various tissues or organs. (3) Increased, decreased or vitiated quantity or quality of waste products.

Symptoms indicate the type of disturbance in the body and gives us guidelines about the treatment. Often the symptom while giving a signal of ill health to the patient, also gives clue to the physician to act appropriately and correct the disturbance of *doshas*, tissues and waste products and restore health. Some of the symptoms, their interpretation and significance is given below.

FEVER

Fever indicates presence of toxins, pyrogens and vitiated *doshas* in the body fluids and blood circulation. During fever, activity of various tissue enzymes increase, which leads to rapid digestion of pyrogens or toxins by various cells in the body fluids.

High body temperature by itself will denature or detoxify the various toxins, which give rise to fever. In addition, the increased activity of various tissues and cellular enzymes, particularly in the white cells, macrophages and reticulo-endothelial cells help to digest the various toxins and pyrogens. The digestive enzymes and appetite are decreased in fever. This helps by cutting down the food intake and further formation of *ama* or toxins. Fever will persist till all the toxins or germs are digested, killed or thrown away from the body. We boil milk and water to destroy the germs. Nature raises body temperature to destroy germs, or denature toxins or *ama* which give rise to fever. Thus fever, like a true friend will not leave the body till the last germ is killed or the body is free from all the toxins.

Doshas and Fever : The character of the fever gives us an idea about the *dosha* which is affected. Irregular fever, high fever and mild fever indicate increase in *Vata, Pitta* and *Kapha doshas* respectively.

Tissues and Fever : The following table gives us the important symptoms seen when particular tisue is affected by toxins :

Tissue affected by toxins of fever	Symptoms
• *Rasa*	Anorexia, vomiting
• *Rakta*	Burning sensation and skin eruptions
• Muscular tissue	Pain or cramps in the calves
• Fatty tissue	Excessive perspiration
• Bony tissue	Pain in the bones
• Norveous tissue	Loss of consciousness

Thus, cramps in the calf muscles indicate that the toxins of fever have entered the muscular tissue and are being digested by the enzymes in t muscles. Thus, one gets lot of information about the affected *doshas* tissues by studying the character of fever and its associated symptoms.

Temperature curves and associated symptoms also give guidelines about the stage of the disease and its prognosis. Thus, fever is a friend of the patient, as it itself acts as a therapeutic agent. Feveris also a friend of physician, as gives the physician important guidelines about the stage of disease, *doshas* and tissues affected, which help him to treat the patient with appropriate measures.

ATISARA

Diarrhoea, i.e. increased frequency of stools with liquid

consistency a symptom of intestinal dysfunction. Diarrhoea occurs because of increased peristalsis of intestines, inflammation of intestines and indigestion of fo because of weak digestive power. Diarrhoea helps the patient by getting rid of undigested food matter and toxins from the intestines.

Character of the stools gives us indication of the affected *doshas* , e.g. reddish and foamy stool with colicky pain is seen in *Vataja* diarrhoea. Watery, yellowish or reddish stools with thrist and burning sensation indicates *Pittaja*, diarrhoea. Whitish, sticky and foul-smelling stools indicate *Kaphaja* diarrhoea.

During early or *ama* stage, the stools are sticky, foul smelling and heavy, i.e. they sink in water. Physician should not attempt to stop diarrhoea during this stage, as the toxins retained in tile intestines can give rise to distension of abdomen, paralytic ileus and if absorbed into circulation may give rise to toxaemia.

Similarly, cough and vomiting help the body to get rid off toxins, bacteria, etc. from the lungs and stomach.

PAIN

Pain indicates dysfunction of a particular organ, forces the patient to see his physician, who otherwise is likely to ignore other minor symptoms. As pain is a late symptom of *prachayatmak* disease, the diagnosis of cancer is often missed for a long time and by the time the patient suffers from pain, the disease has already disseminated and advanced to the incurable stage. Site of the pain indicates the organ affected and character of pain indicates *dosha* responsible for the pain, e.g. acute splitting or pricking unbearable pain is always due to increased or vitiated *Vata*, e.g. the pain of angina pectoris is due to spasm of coronary vessels due to increased *Vata* in the heart. The burning pain indicates increased *Pitta*, while sense of heaviness indicates increased *Kapha*. The time of aggravation of pain, its relation to food and activity and relieving factors give important clues to the physician.

TUMOR

Tumor occurs as a result of collection of molecules or abnormal and excessive growth of cells. Tumor represents an attempt of the body to localise abnormal molecules or cells so that they do not derange the function. If the same abnormal molecules or cells had disseminated all over the body, the disease would have become incurable, progressed fast and diminished the life span of the individual. Lymphosarcoma, a malignant disease can be treated effectively by surgical removal and irradiation. The same lymphosarcoma, when disseminated gives rise to leukemia, which is much more difficult to control and erradicate as the malignant cells are disseminated throughout the body.

The site, character, consistency, etc. of the tumor gives guidelines to the physician about the causative factors, pathogenesis, prognosis and treatment, so that he can treat the patient appropriately. Every individual symptom gives guidelines to the physician about the aetiology.

(i) *Muscle Cramps* **:** This indicate increased *Vata* as a result of excessive exertion or eating diet which is dominant in *Vata* molecules. If dietetic factors are the root cause of cramps, no amount of rest, massage, etc. can help the patient fully. The general treatment of muscle cramps will be directed towards (1) rest, (2) oil massage and wet fomentation, which will neutralise the local *Vata*, (3) the diet predominant in ghee, oil, sour, salty and sweet food items, and (4) muscle tonics like *Karik, ashvagandha, vidarikanda*.

(ii) *Burning Sensation all Over the Body (Sarvangadaha)* **:** This indicate increased molecules of *Pitta* all over the body, which are are affecting blood as well as the nervous tissue (*majja dhatu*). The treatment consists of correcting the root cause, which may be working in the Sun, kitchen or mines for a long time and consuming regularly pungent, sour and salty food items, or psychological factors like anger (increase in *raja* molecules, which in turn increase *Pitta* molecules). The treatment consists of (1) cooling measures like remaining in airconditioned rooms and application of cooling paste of sandalwood, (2) avoiding pungent, sour and salty food items and consumption of sweet and bitter food items, (3) cooling tonics for blood like dried black grapes, dates, *amalaka*, *chandana*, etc., and (4) cooling measures (diet and tonics) for *majja dhatu*, e.g. *kushmanda*, ghee, coconut, *brahmi*, *praval*, etc.

(iii) *Sense of Heavines in the Body* : Heaviness is caused by (a) increase in the weight, i.e. fat, (b) edema, (c) laziness and inactivity, and (d) eating excess of sweet, sour and salty items which will increase *Kapha* molecules.

Treatment : It consists of (i) correcting the root cause, (ii) Advising exercises, (iii) advising diet dominant in pungent and bitter food items avoiding excess of sweet, sour, salty and fatty food items, and (iv) medicines and tonics which decrease the fatty tissue in the body like *haritaki*, Ginger, garlic, Horsegram, *yava*, etc. Even a minor symptoms indicates disturbance in the balanced state of *Vata*, *Pitta*, *Kapha*, tissues or waste products, which is the begining of fhe diease process. If every symptom is scanned and treated appropriately as mentioned above majority of the diseases can be cured. Even in established diseases like *rajayakhsma*, i.e. tuberculosis, *grahani*, i.e. malabsorption, *madhumeha*, i.e. diabetes mellitus, the individual symptoms of every patient suffering from the same disease differ. Each individual symptom give us guidelines to the *dosha*, *dhatu* and *mala* affected and hence the physician should treat all the cases suffering from the same disease in individual manner considering the state of his *doshas*, *dhatus* and *malas*.

14

DEFENCE MECHANISM OF THE BODY
(ROGAPAHARA KSHAMATA)

Every living organism has to adapt and struggle continuously to maintain its structural and functional integrity. At birth, the organism is thrown into an infinite universe and its chance of survival can be compared only to a certain extent with that of a small boat sailing singly in an ocean. Every living creature is continuously being attacked by the five basic elements namely space, wind, energy, water and earth. On the other hand, this little creature tries not only to adapt continuously to the changing environment, but utilises, digests, absorbs and assimilates the same elements and grows and survives on them. In this struggle between the individual and the environment if the individual wins, i.e. controls and utilises the environment in a masterly manner, he enjoys sound health. If the individual cannot face the environment in an effective manner, but continues to struggle and survive, he suffers from a disease. On the other hand if environment wins, death ensues. Thus, health or disease is the result of interplay of resistance of the individual and environment.

Man has to constantly adjust to the continuously changing environment, e.g. temperature, humidity, breeze, etc. which vary from time to time, from day to day and from season to season. Man has developed some control over environment, e.g. by using air-conditioners and hearing devices he can still maintain comfortable ambient temperature. Ayurveda has outlined daily and seasonal regimen so that one can withstand daily and seasonal changes in the environment easily and one doesn't become a prey to the disease.

Every individual is born with a specific constitution, which he inherits from his parents. A person with healthy genes has an ideal constitution, which can resist various stresses and strains in life easily. More the defective genes, worse is the constitution. Such a person suffers from severe diseases and dies a premature death. The constitution, i.e. resistance is constantly modified by diet, rest, activity, happiness, sorrow and environmental factors.

In Ayurved defence mechanism, i.e. resistance at various levels is described as follows :

(1) Relative proportion of the causal elements, i.e. *sattva, raja* and *tama* in mind. Persons with predominance of *tama* element are unable to tolerate even slight pain and break down under ordinary stresses and strains of life. Person with predominance of *raja* elements get emotionally upset over trivial matters and are prone to emotional outbursts and temper tantrums. Persons with predominance of *sattva* element can withstand extra ordinary stresses and strains of life without difficulty, A *tamas* person never takes decisions. *Rajasa* persons are likely to take wrong decisions, whereas *sattvik* person always take right decisions even under condition of stress.

These decisions constitute most vital defence mechanism of the body, on these decisions depend even the survival of the individual. *Prajnaparadha,* i.e. not following one's conscience is the root cause of all the diseases. For increasing *sattva guna,* i.e. for strengthening the mind and avoiding psychosomatic disorders one should follow : (i) the rules of good conduct at activity, and (ii) suppress various desires, instincts and emotions and develop philosophical attitude towards life.

(2) A Relative proportion of five basic elements in the body, i.e. space, air, energy, water and earth. Health may be defined as a state of perfect balance between the five, basic elements both quantitatively and qualitatively. Increase or decrease in any element gives rise to disease and lowered resistance of the body, e.g. decreased and increased water content of the body give rise to dehydration and oedema respectively. Increase or decrease in

internal enerl gives rise to fever and shock state respectively. Body offers best resistance when all the basic elements are in balanced state.

(3) Relative proportion of biological molecule, viz. *Vata, Pitta* and *Kapha* molecules constitute the structual and functional units the body which depend all the life process. The unbalanced state these molecules give rise to disease, while the balanced state both quantitatively and qualitatively is defined as health. Persons with *Vata, Pitta* and *Kapha* constitution, e.g. person with *Kapha* constitution feels chilled when exposed to rain, air-conditioned room and may develop cold, coue or an asthmatic attack. Person with *Pitta* constitution is prone develop bleeding disorders if he takes excess of pungent and sour food items or is exposed to sun. On the other hand, a person with balanced constitution rarely suffer from disease and enjoys burning heat of summer biting cold of winter and lashing torrents of monsoon equally well.

How to maintain balanced state of *Vata, Pitta* and *Kadha* and thus prevent disease is given in detail on pages 137 and 138 of the book, Basic Principl of Ayurveda by the same Author.

(4) Tissues and organs of good qualities. Tissues of inferior qualities are vulnerable to various stresses and strains, e.g. a person of poor quality of muscular tissue is prone to frequent attacks of cold. A person with inherited defect in the synthesis of blood may suffer from diseases like Cooley's anaemia for which there is no cure. On the other hand a person with good quality of liver and heart rarely suffer from an attack of jaundice and heart attack respectively.

A person with poor quality of bones is prone to develop fractures even with slight injury. On the other hand, a person with good quality of tissues rarely develops disease related to that tissue, e.g. person with ideal nervous tissue will rarely develop an attack of poliomyelitis, meningitis, etc. and will have intact memory even at the age of 100 years.

The resistance of the tissues is improved by administering

appropriate diet and tissue tonics as advised in chapter fifteen of Basic principles of Ayurveda and in the chapter on *Rasayana,* i.e. tonics.

In addition, Ayurveda has also mentioned diet and medicines which act as tonics for various organs, e.g. *hridya* diet and medicine means diet and medicine which act as tonic for heart. Similarly, *netrya* means eye tonics, *keshya* means hair tonic, *kanthya* means throat tonics, etc.

Thus, healthy molecules, tissues and organs which have ideal structure and functions can defend themselves as well as the body from various stresses and strains of life.

रोगापहारक्षमता

दहधातुप्रत्यनीकभूतानि द्रव्याणि देहधातुभिर्विरोधमापद्यन्ते ।   (च. सू. 26/81)

व्याधिक्षमत्वं व्याधिबलविरोधित्वं व्याध्युत्पाद् प्रतिबन्धकत्वम् इति ।

(चक्रपाणि)

(रोगविज्ञान तथा विकृति विज्ञान- रानडे पृ. 42.)

शरीराणि चातिस्थूलान्यतिकृशान्यनिविष्टमांसशोणितास्थीनि दुर्बलान्यसात्म्या-
हारोपचितान्यल्पाहाराण्यल्पसत्त्वानि च भवन्त्यव्याधिसहानि, विपरीतानि
पुनर्व्याधिसहानि ।   (च. सू. 28/7)

(रोगविज्ञान-विकृति विज्ञान-रानडे-पृ. 42)

15

ROOT CAUSES OF DISEASE
(ROGANAM MULAKARANANI)

The imbalanced state of *doshas*, i. e. structural and functional molecules (both intracellular as well as extracellular) of the body, *dhatus* and *malas* is defined as disease. The various aetiological factors alter the milieu interior, i.e. bring about quantitative increase or decrease, or alter quality of the various *doshas*, *dhatus* and *malas*. The aetiological factors as well as precipitating factors are limited. The same aetiological factor can give rise to number of diseases or different diseases in different persons, e.g. indigestion may give rise to rheumatism, bronchial asthma, skin disorders or vomiting and diarrhoea depending on which organ is weak in a particular patient. The products of indigestion, i.e. *ama* gets absorbed in circulation and accumulate in tissues or organs which can't resist their entry. Weakness of tissues or organs is either hereditary, i.e. genetic in origin or is the result of various illnesses or insults. A person with weak lungs is susceptible to recurrent attacks of cough or asthma, while a person with weak intestines suffers from recurrent attacks of diarrhoea and dysentery. In a person with marked weakness of a particular organ, the disease will be precipitated by minor or insignificant precipitating factors, e.g. even exposure to breeze or fan, fatigue, infection, hair bath, etc. can precipitate an attack of asthma in a persoin born with weak lungs. A person born with genetically healthy tissues can live a full life of over hundred years inspite of all the vices and irregularities of life, On the other hand, one peg of alcohol or smoking few cigarettes may cause cirrhosis of liver or lung cancer in persons with weak liver and lungs respectively.

In medicine, vary rarely can we incriminate one agent as

the cause of a disease. Even in case of infectious disease causative organism is only one ol the causes of the disease, e.g. though we say that poliomyelitis is caused by virus of polio, only one out of five thousand cases infected with the virus develop an attack of paralysis in poliomyelitis. Only those children whose nervous tissue can't defend itself against polio virus develop poliomyelitis. The susceptibility to the disease is increased by injury, exertion and fatigue. Thus, poliomyelitis is caused by not the virus of polio alone but by number of factors like, (i) inherent weakness of anterior horn cells, (ii) poor defence mechanism of the body like antibody formation, (iii) lower resistance of the anterior born cells by factors like injury, exertion, fatigue, injection, etc. (iv) the number of polio viruses entering in the body, (v) virulence of polio virus, and (vi) state of immunity of the child which may be natural following previous exposure to the virus or acquired as a result of administration of polio vaccine. Thus, every disease is multi-factorial in origin, though some factors may be more important than others as causative agents.

The details of history gives clue to the aetiological factors, which include the main causative factors as well as the aggravating, relieving and precipitating factors. Examination of the patient as well as the history give us an idea about the structural and functional state of various biological molecules, i.e. *Vata*, *Pitta* and *Kapha* various tissues and organs and waste products.

It is much more important to understand the genesis of the symptom, or the disease process in an individual patient rather than labelling the name of the disease. This is natural as unless the aetiological factors which vary from patient to patient are corrected, the disease cannot be eradicated, e.g. treating lung cancer alone is not sufficient unless one tackles the route cause, i.e. smoking. Hence, the physician who understands aetiopathogenesis of the diseases can alone got the insight into the disease process and guide the patient correctly so that he can restore his health.

11
AYURVEDIC RECIPES
AND THEIR PREPARATIONS

Ayurvedic medicines are prepared from plants, animals, metals like gold, iron, minerals, *ksharas* or by combination of plants and minerals or metals. Eight parts of the plants namely leaves, flowers, fruits, skin, branches, trunk, roots and the gums are used for preparation of medicines. The part of the plant which contains maximum quantity of the substance having medicinal property is used.

General rules which give guidelines as to which part of the plant should be used.

  (i) If the roots are large, their skin should be taken. If the root is small the entire root should be taken.

 (ii) In banyan and *jamun* trees, the skin of the trunk should be used, while in *khadira*, i.e. catechu tree and *asana* tree the central portion of the trunk should be used.

(iii) The leaves of *tamala jalisa*, *nagavalli* (betel leaves) and *nimba* tree should be used.

(iv) Fruits of *aamalaka*, *bibhitaka* and *haritaki* should be used.

 (v) Flowers of *palasha, dhataki* and rose should be used.

(vi) The milky juice of *arka* and cactus should be used. After taking out, the part of the herb should be preserved well in a clean jar and protected from sun, rain, humidity, dust and insects.

Juice, *kalka, hima,* decoction, *pant,* medicated water and medicated milk should always be taken fresh.

After drying, the medicinal properties are retained upto one year. The dry parts of the plants should not be used as medicine after one year. The expiry date of various Ayurvedic medicinal recipes are given in the following table :

Recipe	Expiry Date
Churna (Powder)	4 months
Arka	4 months
Medicated Oil and Ghee	6 months
Tablets, *Avaleha* and *Prasha*	1 year
Arishta, Asava	3 years
Bhasmas of Metals	3 years

PURIFICATION OF MEDICINES

Medicines are purified to reduce their harmful effects a follows : (i) *Arjuna is* boiled in milk, (ii) Garlic, marking nut, *jayaphala* and *bachanaga* are boiled in milk, (iii) *Hingul is* triturated in juice of garlic, and (iv) *Tamra bhasma* (copper oxide) is triturated in juice of *kumari* or *tulsi.*

Medicines having similar properties are used in decoction powders and other recipes to reduce the dose and the side effects of single medicine.

Medicines having opposite properties are sometimes used to reduce the side effects, e.g. seeds of *jayaphala* are laxative and give rise to colicky pain.

By triturating the seeds of *jayaphala* in lemon juice, the colicky pain does not occur.

MEDICINAL RECIPES OF HERBS

It is always better to use fresh plants. However, every plant is not available everywhere and fruits and flowers of all plants are available only in a particular season. Hence, various recipes are prepared which retain the medicinal active ingredient for a longer period.

Fresh medicines are dried and given in powder form. If the

active ingredient is¹ soluble in hot water, the decoction is given. If the active ingredient dissolves in hot water but is destroyed by prolonged heating *phant* is given. If the active ingredient is destroyed by heat *hima,* i.e. *shita is* given. If the active ingredient evaporates then *arka is* given.

If the active ingredient is soluble in alcohol, then *asava* or *arishta is* given.

Sneha, avaleha and *prasha* are prepared by boiling the medicine with jaggery or sugar solution till the water evaporates. The plants are burnt to get the minerals and *ksharas.*

The gum like secretions of trees maintain their medicinal properties for a long time.

PROPORTION OF MEDICINES IN A RECIPE

Whenever many medicines constitute ingredients of a medical recipe like decoction, powder, medicated ghee etc., and their proportion or quantity is not mentioned, the ingredients should be taken in equal proportion while preparing the recipe.

(i) *Svarasa* : Fresh plants should be grinded in mortar and pestle or in a mixer. The pulp should be kept in a clean thin cotton bag. The bag should be squeezed and the juice extracted. This fresh juice is known as *svarasa.*

Guduchi, nimba and *vasa* contain more fibres. Hence, it is not easy to obtain fresh juice. In these cases the part of the plant should be steamed in a cooker and later the juice should be extracted. The *svarasa,* i.e. fresh juice is easily absorbed and its effects are seen in a short time.

Dose : 20 ml., i.e. 4 teaspoonfuls twice a day.

Fresh juice should be given in morning and evening. *Svarasa* is usually given with honey, jaggery, sugar, *saindhava,* salt, cumin seeds or ghee.

(ii) *Kalka (Chatni)* : The pulp of fresh part of the plant prepared by grinding is known as *kalka. Svarasa* contains only the liquid elements. *Kalka* contains both the solid as well as the liquid ingredients of the plant. *Kalka is* more ofter used for external application. Internally it should be taken fresh.

Dose : 10 grams, i.e. 2 teaspoonfuls.

(iii) *Quath (Decoction)* : Boiling with water a single or many medicinal plants till one quarter or one eighth of original quantity of water remains is known as decoction. Fresh parts of plant to be used as medicine should be soaked in water for 12 hours. Depending on whether the part of the plant is brittle, semihard or hard, water should be added in quantity which is four times, eight times or sixteen times the quantity of the part of the plant respectively and boiled till one quarter of the original amount of water remains.

In case the dried plants are used, depending on whether the plant is brittle, semihard or hard. Water should be added in quantity which is eight times, sixteen times or thirty two times the quantity of the dry plant respectively and boiled till one eighth of the original amount of water remains.

This decoction should be used fresh or at the most within one hour of its preparation.

Precautions to be taken while preparing decoction :

(a) Decoction should not be made if the plant is fragrant,

(b) While boiling do not cover the vessel with a dish, and

(c) The flame used should be of low intensity just to keep the decoction boiling.

In *vataja, pittaja* and *kaphaja* diseases, sugar should be added in quantity which is one : sixth, one : fourth and one : sixteenth of the powder or the fresh part of the plant used respectively.

Dose : 40 grams, i.e. 40 ml., or eight teaspoonfuls morning and evening on empty stomach.

(iv) *Kshirapaka (Medicated milk)* : Medicated milk is prepared by boiling together one part of juice or powder of the plant, four parts of cow's milk and thirty two parts of water till the water evaporates. The medicated milk is useful in chronic fever and stomach-ache.

The penetrating hot, pungent and astringent qualities of the medicines are subdued in medicated milk. One should not use medicines with sour or salty tastes as the milk will split. The medicated milk should not be used in initial or *aama* stage of the disease. It should be used in *pakva* stage of the disease and in chronic diseases.

(v) **Shadangodaka (Medicated water)** : It is used in fever, to be taken frequently in small quantity to reduce the fever and quench the thirst.

Musta, parpataka ushira, white sandalwood, red sandalwood and ginger are the medicines used in equal quantity in *shadangodaka*. It is prepared by boiling together one part of the mixture of powders of these medicines in one hundred twenty eight parts of water till half the quantity of water remains.

(vi) **Hima or Shita** : This recipe is used to preserve the active ingredients in sticky fragrant plants with cold quality.

Powder the plants with above quantities. Soak one part of the powder in six parts of water for twelve hours. After straning, the *hima* should be taken. It is useful in burning sensation and getting rid of foul smell of body or discharges. It is useful in *pittaja* diseases.

Dose : 80 ml.

If necessary honey or sugar should be added. It should be taken in the morning on empty stomach.

(vii) **Mantha** : *Mantha is* the recipe prepared by churning the liquid medicinal preparation.

40 gm., of the plant medicines and 160 ml. of water should be well mixed and churned in a mixer. Later it should be strained and taken.

(viii) **Phant** : When the active ingredient is soluble in hot water but destroyed by prolonged heating. *Phant* preparation is useful.

One part of the powder of the medicine or fresh medicine should be kept in a vessel and four parts of boiling water should be poured and a dish should be kept as a cover over the vessel till the preparation becomes warm. Later it should be strained and taken. This process is the same as used in preparation of tea.

Dose : 80 ml.

Depending on *dosha,* ghee, jaggery or sugar should be added to *Phant.*

(ix) ***Churna (Powder) :*** The dry medicines are powdered. It is used for preparing decoction of the medicine. It can be used for external massage and preparing other recipes.

Churna, i.e. powder should be taken with *anupana.* i.e. adjuvant.

Powder	Adjuvant	Dose of Adjuvant
One Part	Jaggery	Two parts
One Part	Sugar	Two parts
One Part	Oil or Gee	Two parts
One Part	Milk	Four parts

Dose : Powder of only one plant-5 grams.

A mixture of powders of many medicines-10 grams.

Tablets are prepared by boiling powder with jaggerya or sugar solution in water till water evaporates.

(x) ***Satva :*** The white starchy ingredient of plants, tubers, grains is known as *satva.*

Guduchi satva : The stem of guduchi should be grinded in water and kept in it. The starchy substance collects at bottom. The supernatant water should be gently removed by a ringe. The solid portion at the bottom should be spread in a dish and dried. The white powder is known as *satva.*

Dose : 250 to 500 ml./grams.

(xi) ***Avaleha :*** A*valehas* are the medicinal recipes prepared by boiling the indicated herbs in decoction form in solutions of sugar or jaggery till they attain the consistency of honey. *Avalehas* are licked.

Avaleha are prepared so that : (a) Medicines become durable, (b) The taste of the medicine becomes sweet, and (c) The nutritional value increases because of jaggery or sugar.

(i) *Preparation of decoction* : Take the indicated herb or herbs. Depending on the consistency, i.e. whether it is brittle, semi-hard or hard, add water in quantity of eight, sixteen, or thirtytwo times that of herbal medicine. Boil till one quarter or one eighth part remains in the form of decoction.

(ii) *Adding jaggery or sugar*: Add jaggery or sugar dissolved in water to the decoction and boil on low flame. Add four teaspoonfuls of milk while boiling. After boiling, the blackish waste floats on water which should be removed.

Depending on consistency, the recipe is called :

(a) *Tantupaka* : In which when the spoon is dipped and taken away slowly for one or two inches, a band of the recipe is seen between the recipes and the spoon.

(b) *Bindupaka* : If a small portion of the recipe is poured on a dish, it assumes the form of a round pill. In *bindupaka* the amount of water is less compared to that in *tantupaka*.

PRAKSHEPANA MEDICINES

Depending on the disease other herbal medicines are added in the form of fine powder to *tantupaka* or *bindupaka* while it is hot and stirred well. Powders of the fragrant herbs should be added after the recipe is cool. At the end, honey should be added. Honey should never be added to the hot recipe.

Depending on consistency, *avaleha is* of two types, semisolid and solid.

The following tests confirms that the *avaleha is* well prepared and will be durable : (i) *Avaleha* sticks to finger and forms a thin bard when the finger is slowly taken away, (ii)

Avaleha sinks in water and does not dissolve, (iii) When pressed with fingers the lines on finger are seen clearly, and (iv) The colour and smell of the *Avaleha* is the same as those of medicines used in preparation of *avaleha*.

Dose : 40 gm.

Avaleha should be taken as such. No adjuvants are necessary. Milk may be used as an adjuvant.

Expiry date : One year.

Uses of Avalehas : (i) As medicines, e.g. *vasavaleha* in cough, *(ii) Rasayana :* Tissue tonic, e.g. *chyavanaprasha avaleha*, and (iii) Adjuvant : K*antakari avaleha* is used along with medicines used for cough.

In general medicinal herbs, jaggery or sugar, water, honey and gee are used in the preparation of *avaleha*.

Depending on consistency it is classified as : (i) *Leha*-semisolid and licked, (ii) *Avaleha*-more solid and licked, (iii) *Prasha*-solid it has to be bitten, e.g. *cyavanaprasha*.

Paka : *Paka* of garlic or *kushmanda*, i.e. asha-gourd (*petha*) *kushmanda paka*.

One kilogram of pulp of *kushamanda,* 160 grams of ghee and one kg. of sugar should be boiled over low flame till water evaporates. While it is hot, add 20 grams each of *pippali*, ginger and cumin seeds and five grams each of *temalapatra*, cardamom, coriander and pepper. Spread over a dish and cut into pieces of ten grams each.

Dose : 10 to 20 grams.

It is nutritious and strengthening.

(xii) *Arks :* *Arka* means sun. Liquid recipe which contains powerful active ingredient is called *arks*. The volatile substances in the herbs are lost in air while boiling. These active ingredients can be preserved in water by process of distillation. These volatile substances have a tendency to vaporise. Hence, *arka* should be preserved in air tight bottles. Even then they are gradually lost.

Hence, *arka* should be used within six months of its manufacturing date. Depending on the smell on the volatile substances *arka* may be with good smell, bad smell or without any smell.

Dose : 10 to 40 ml.

Arka of *ajamoda* and fennel seeds are used in indigestion, gases, pain in abdomen, etc.

(xiii) ***Asava and Arishta* :** Active ingrdients in some herbs are soluble in alcohol. *Asava is* prepared by fermenting fresh juice. *Arishta* is prepared by fermenting decoction.

Asava and *arashta* are prepared as follows :

Mix the following ingredients—(a) Fresh juice of herbs for *asava* and decoction of herbs for *arishta,* (b) Jaggery, honey, sugar which undergo fermentation easily, (c) *Dhataki* flowers as they contain yeast cells which help fermentation, (d) Fragrant drugs like camphor, *jatamansi.*

Mix the above four and keep them in a vessel at a particular temperature for fifteen to thirty days. After fifteen days clear, transparent *asava* or *arishta* with attractive colour and smell is ready for use.

Dose : 10 to 50 ml.

Asava and *arishta* are used for treatment of diseases and as general tonics. All *asavas* and *arishtas* are hot and increase *pitta.* Hence, they are contrain-dicated in *pittaja* diseases, ulcer, acidity, jaundice, diseases of liver and bleeding disorders.

Asava and *arishta* are light, minute, pentrating and hot and stimulate the body and mind. They increase the digestive power and are useful in diseases with dominatnt *kapha dosha.*

(xiv) ***Medicated oil and ghee* :** One part of the grinded fresh herbs or powders of dry herbs, four parts of *tila* oil or ghee and sixteen parts of decoction of the same herbs should be boiled over low fire till the water evaporates. This is called as medicated oil or ghee.

Tests to know that the medicated oil or ghee is well prepared.

(a) When the foam appears while the medicated oil is boiling, it is ready for use, (b) When the foam disappears while the medicated ghee is boiling, it is ready for use, (c) When a few drops of medicated oil or ghee are poured on fire, it produce noise and smoke if some water is still remaining. When the entire water has evaporated, putting the drops of oil or ghee on flame or fire wilt not produce any noise or smoke, (d) The colour, taste and smell of the medicated herbs should be present in the medicated oil or ghee, and (e) If you can preapre a wick from the *kalka of* herbs in medicated oil or ghee, it is ready for use.

Snehapaka : When the medicated oil or ghee is prepared, the qualities depend on how long it is boiled. Depending on the duration of boiling, it is classified as—(i) *Mridu paka* : Soft consistency because all the water has not evaporated. (ii) *Madhya paka* : Medium consistency because all the water has evaporated as advised in *avaleha, (iii) Khara paka* : Hard consistency beeuase the boiling continues even after all the water has evaporated. It develops a blackish colour.

Uses : (i) *Kharapaka* should be used for external massage, (ii) *Mridupaka* should be used for preparing nose drops, and (iii) *Madhyamapaka is* used as medicine by mouth. *Avaleha is* also used for giving enema.

Advantages : (i) In medicated oil or ghee the ingredients soluble in water as well as oil are present, (ii) *Avaleha* can be used for one year after it's manufactured, (iii) Because of boiling, the medicine is easily digested, (iv) Medicated oil is used internally as medicine and can be used for oil massage, (v) Because of oil and ghee, the medicines act as nourishing agent, subdue *vata* and help in healing of wounds.

Dose : 10 to 40 ml.

It should be taken with warm water.

(xv) *Guggul* : Guggul is the natural gum which oozes from the skin of trunk of tree during winter and summer. Depending on the tree from which guggul is collected, the qualities differ.

General qualites of guggul : (a) It is laxative and hence subdues pitta, (b) It is hot and therefore subdues *vata* and *kapha,* (c) It stimulates digestive power and purifies ducts, (d) It improves qualities of tissues and acts as *rasayana,* (e) It helps to get rid of foul smell of gases and discharges.

Purification of guggul : The guggul naturally removed from the tree contains earth, dust, etc. which stick to it. Remove the small stones, earth, etc. which are obviously seen. Later the *guggul* should be kept in a thin cotton bag and the cotton bag kept in decoction of *triphala* or *dashamula* which is kept boiling on a low flame. This process purifies *guggul.*

The methods to prepare medicated *guggul* :

(a) *Soma Paka* : The indicated medicines are triturated with *guggul* and later tablets or rounded pills are prepared.

(b) *Surya Paka* : The powder of *guggul* should be dissolved in liquid preparation of herbs, e.g. decoction, *phant, hima* and dried in hot sun. Repeat the process 21 times and prepare tablets.

(c) *Anala paka* : *Guggul* is heated on a low flame and later tablets or pills prepared.

The recipes which contain at least 50 % *guggul* are called as *guggul kalpa.*

Guggul preparations are useful not only in *vataja* diseases, but also in *pittaja* as well as *kaphaja* diseases.

Dose : 240 mgms.

(xvi) *Mashi* : Black ash of any substance is called *mashi.* When a substance is burnt halfway, the ash is black. If it is burnt fully the ash is white.

The black ash contains coal :

(a) *Hastidanta mashi* : Black ash of elephant's tooth. It is allied externally for baldness.

(b) *Mayurapichchha Mashi* : The black ash of peacock's feather and equal part of powder of *pippali* should be mixed and licked off and on with honey. It is useful in hiccough, vomiting and breathlessness.

(xvii) *Kshara* : Three types of *ksharas* are used in Ayurveda :

(a) Natural *kshara* as available in mines, e.g. *Sajji kshara* (Sodium carbonate), *Souvarchala* (Potassium nitrate), *Tankana kshara* (Sodium borate).

These *ksharas* can be prepared in laboratory.

(b) Ksharas prepared from herbs. The entire plant is burnt till white ash remains. The ash should be kept in an earthen pot and four times its quantity of water is added. The mixture is stirrred and kept for twelve hours in the earthen pot. The supernatant fluid should be removed and boiled on a low flame. The *Kshara* collects at the bottom.

(c) *Ksharas* prepared from animal products, e.g. *navasagrara*, i.e. Ammonium chloride is prepared from urine of animals.

Qualites and uses of ksharas : (a) *Kshara* is pungent,hot and penetrating, (b) It is useful for ripening of abscess because of dominant fire element, (c) It is useful to get rid of excessive granulation tissue in an ulcer, (d) It is harmful to generative tissue and semen, (e) *Kshara sutra* is used for chemical cautery of fistula.

Dose : 120 to 240 mgms.

It is given with milk or ghee.

(xviii) *Preparation of metals* : For thousands of years, herbal medicines are use in Ayurveda by *Rishis*. Hence, the use of herbal medicines is know as *arshasampradaya*.

In the first century Nagarjuna used mercury *(rasa)* and various preparation of metals *(dhatu)* in treatment of diseases. Hence, this system is known as *rasa-vidya* or *dhatu-vidya* and the physicians who followed this system are known as belonging to *siddha sampradaya*.

Iron and Calcium are important ingredients of red blood cells and bones respectively. In addition copper, iodine, cobalt, fluorine, magnesium and zinc are present in minute quantities in body. If the quantity of these elements is decreased in the body their deficiency symptoms are seen. If their quantity increase in body their side effects are seen.

The preparations of metals are not easily assimilated by the body. Hence, they are given in small amounts as medicines. The metallic preparation, once absorbed are not easily excreted from the body and hence can give rise to long term side effects. The organs affects are blood, nervous systems, kidneys, bone marrow, liver, skin and intestines.

Dose of metallic preparations oxides of metals and precious stones is 30 to 120 mgms. per day. They should not be used for more than four to six weeks.

Tests to see that the oxides, i.e. *bhasma of* metals are of good quality :

(a) It floats on water, (b) When taken in a pinch, the natural lines on finger tips become more obvious, (c) It is smooth and does not have the shine of the metal, (d) If heated in fire, no smoke is sin.

Dose : 30 to 120 mgms.

(xix) *Food preparations* : Rice should be pounded till small granules are formed. These granules are heated over a drying pan. The following preparations are used :

(a) *Manda* : One part of rice granules are cooked in fourteen parts of water. The cooked mixture should be strained over cloth. It should not contain any particles. This is called *manda*. Ginger and saindhava salt are added to *manda* and it is drunk.

(b) *Peya* : One part of rice granules should be cooked in fourteen parts or six parts of water for a longer time till it is thicker manda. A few rice granules are allowed.

(c) *Vilepi* : One part of rice granules should be cooked in four parts of water till a thick *kanji* with particles is formed.

(d) *Tandulodaka (Rice washing)* : One part of rice should be mixed with eight parts of water and the mixture stirred with hands and kept as such for six hours. The mixture should be strained and the whitish rice washings are used in treatment of diarrhoea and excessive white vaginal discharge.

(e) *Manda of rice popcorn* : One part of powder of rice popcorn should be boiled in fourteen parts of water. This *manda is* useful in diarrhoea, malabsorption and fever.

(f) *Yusha (Soup of pulses)* : (i) Amongst pulses like *mung, masur, tur, udid* and *Chana* and appropriate *dal,* i.e. pulse should be selected. Forty grams of the pulse, forty grams of pulp *(kalka)* of approrpiate medicinal herbs and five grams each of ginger and *pippali* should be cooked in 640 ml. of water. The mixture should be strained and drunk.

(ii) General yush (Soup) : Twenty grams each of rice, *mung dal, udid dal* and *tila* (Sesame seeds) should be cooked in 360 ml. of water. This soup should be taken by mouth. It is used during recovery stage of fever.

(iii) Kulatha soup : One part each of *kulattha, yava, badara, mung, radish* and ginger should be boiled in sixteen parts of water, and drunk.

(iv) Khichadi (Krishara) : Soft *khichadi* prepared by boiling a mixture of rice, tila and *udid,* subdues *vata* but increases *pitta* and *kapha.*

(v) Vesavara (Mutton soup) : The pieces of meat of goat with fat removed should be crushed and cooked after adding ginger, pepper, *pippali,* jaggery and ghee. This soup is nourishing and increase the strength.

(g) *Madya (Alcoholic drinks)* : Types of Alcoholic drinks

(i) Sidhu : The alcohol drink prepared from fermentation of juices of sugarcane, pomegranate or grapes in know as *sidhu.*

(ii) Varuni : The alcoholic drink prepared from fermentation of juice oozing from the trunk of trees of dates, coconut or tadi is called *varuni,* e.g. *nira, toddy.*

(iii) Sura : The alcoholic drink prepared from fermentation of cereals like rice, wheat, yava is called *sura.*

These alcoholic drinks are not used as medicines. *Asava* and *arishta* are used as medicines.

EXTERNAL APPLICATION

Application of *lepa*, i.e. paste of medicines is useful in cases of pain, oedema or discolouration of skin. For a wound, or an ulcer an ointment is applied. Poultice is applied for ripening of an abscess or liquefaction of pus or phlegm accumulated in chest. The action of *leps*, ointment and *upanaha* continues three hours, five hours and six hours respectively. Later a fresh application should be used. The thickness of paste should be one to two centimeters while the thickness of ointment and poultice should be two to three centimenters.

If itching, oedema, redness or rash appears on application of paste, ointment or poultice it should not be used again.

Fresh herbs should be grinded and their pulp, i.e. *kalka* should be applied externally. The powder of dry herbs should be triturated in water, cow's urine, milk, oil or ghee and applied as a paste.

After use, the paste, ointment or the poultice should be gently removed by cotton dipped in hot water.

Malahara (Ointment) : In *lepa*, the water content is more while the water content is less in ointment. Ointment is prepared by triturating one part of pulp of fresh medicines or powders of dry medicine with *shatadhouta ghrita,* wax, *tila* oil, coconut oil, vaseline or cream.

Upanaha (Poultice) : (i) General poultice-It is prepared by cooking together, powders of *atasi, yava* and wheat, *kanji,* water, cow's urine, *haridra, daruharidra, saindhava* salt and *tila* oil. It should be applied while hot.

(ii) *Atasi* poultice-A mixture of forty grams of *atasi* powder, five grams of ghee, 80 ml. of milk and 2.5 grams of turmeric should be cooked together and the hot pulp placed in thin cotton bag and applied over the affected part.

Uses : (i) For fomentation, (ii) For induction of local sweating., (iii) For relieving pain, (iv) For stiffness of parts, (v) For ripening of an abscess.

SHATADHAUTA GHRITA

Shatadhauta ghrita literally means ghee which is washed one hundred times. Cow's ghee should be mixed with water till the ghee is immersed in water. The mixture should be triturated in a copper vessel. When the water loses its clarity, it should be thrown away. Fresh clean water should added to the ghee and the process repeated hundred times. The ghee becomes softer than that of butter. This ghee is useful in burning sensation in ulcer and for healing of ulcer.

How long should a medicine be administered?

In acute illnesses like cold, cough, vomiting, diarrhoea, the medicines should be given for eight to ten days. In chronic diseases like rheumatism, nephrotic syndrome, the herbal medicines should be used for four to six weeks. If medicines do not relieve the symptoms, reassess the patient and change the medicines.

Metalic preparations should not be used for more than two weeks at a time.

The table on the next page gives the dose, expiry date and adjuvants used for various Ayurvedic recipes :

S. No.	Medicinal Recipe	Dose	Expiry date	Adjuvants
•	Fresh Juice	20 ml., i.e 4 teaspoonfuls	Within one year	Honey, Sugar, Jaggery.
•	Kalka-Pulp	10 grams, i.e. 2 teaspoonfuls	Fresh quantity	Saindhava, Cumin seeds and Ghee
•	Decoction-Kvath	40 ml., i.e. 8 teaspoonfuls	Fresh	(i) Milk and Jaggery in equal (ii) Honey, Ghee and Oil twice the quantity of Kalka Vata diseases 1/6th Sugar quantity of Churna pitta diseases 1/4th Sugar quantity of churna kapha diseases 1/16th Sugar quantity of churna
•	Kshira paka medicated milk	40 to 80 ml.	3 hours	Don't use in early, i.e. aama stage of the disease
•	Medicated water	Fretuently as much as necessary	12 hours	In fever take frequently
•	Hima-Shita	80 ml.	4 to 6 hours	With honey and Sugar
•	Mantha	80 ml.	4 to 6 hours	With honey and Sugar
•	Phant	80 ml.	3 hours	Ghee, Jaggery, Sugar
•	Satva	250 to 500 mg.	3 months	Milk
•	Avaleha	40 grams	1 years	

S.No.	Medicinal Recipe	Dose	Expiry date	Adjuvants
•	*Arka*	10 to 40 ml.	4 months	
•	*Asava* and *Arishta*	10 to 50 ml.	2 to 3 years	
•	Medicated oil and Ghee	5 to 20 mi.	6 months	
•	*Guggul*	250 mg.	1 year	
•	*Mashi*	5 grams	1 year	With honey
•	*Kshara*	120 to 240 mgm.	1 year	With milk or ghee
•	*Bhasma-ash*, i.e. oxides of metals and precious stones	30 to 120 mg.	3 years	